ESSENTIAL OILS FOR ANIMALS

A complete guide to animal wellness using essential oils,
hydrosols and herbal oils

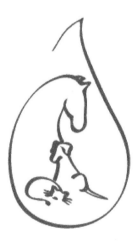

NAYANA MORAG

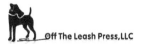

Off The Leash Press, LLC

This book is intended as a guide for anyone who cares for animals and would like to use essential oils and other aromatic extracts in the routine management of health and well-being. It is in no way intended to replace regular veterinary care of your animal, nor is it intended to offer diagnosis, advice or treatment. Please consult with your veterinarian for diagnosis and possible treatment if you are concerned about your pet's health. The author and publisher assume no liability in connection with use of the information presented in this book.

Published by:

Off The Leash Press, LLC,

119 Lucky Dog Lane, Hendersonville, NC 28792

www.offtheleashpress.com

407-758-8309

Second edition

Edited by Robin Moulsdale

Cover design © 2019 Bogdan Matei

All interior photographs property of Nayana Morag.

ISBN 978-0-9841982-9-0

To all those who have shone light on my path

CONTENTS

CONTENTS

ACKNOWLEDGEMENTS

For this second edition my greatest thanks go to all those of you who have taken the time to let me know that you enjoyed the book and have found it useful. You are my inspiration. Apart from that my thanks still go to those of have taught me, particularly Caroline Ingraham, with whom I trained and who pioneered the method of animal self-selection of essential oils. Gabriel Mojay has also been a primary inspiration and teacher. Gabriel's combination of essential oils and Traditional Chinese Medicine took my work to a different level, and his book, "Aromatherapy for Healing the Spirit" is a major reference resource for me. Peter Allan, acupuncturist and dear friend, has also helped me clarify and refine my understanding of the Five Element Theory, and continues to do so whenever we have an extra couple of hours to spend on the phone.

This book would not have come into being without my father Robin Moulsdale who gave me the ability to write coherently in the first place, much good advice on style and content on the first draft of this book, plus a lifetime of support and encouragement. Many thanks also to Sherri Cappabianca from Off The Leash Press, whose collaboration with this project has been beyond invaluable, may we see many more books unleashed.

Thanks to all my students and colleagues who contributed case studies for inclusion in the book. Thank you for sharing this journey, helping me learn through teaching, and inspiring me with your enthusiasm.

Heart-felt thanks to my partner Prasado. He has been supportive in so many ways that I can't even start to list them, so I shan't. But this book would not exist without his encouragement and in-put, and his cooking.

And leaving the best for last (which is also how I eat my food), I thank all the animals who have taught me so much. I have never met an animal who didn't have something to teach me, but I am especially grateful to all the redheads (cats and horses) who have blessed my life and made me laugh, and to Gipsy, sweet soul and wise teacher, who is always with me. And to the new generation of fur friends who bring me joy daily and make sure I never stand still.

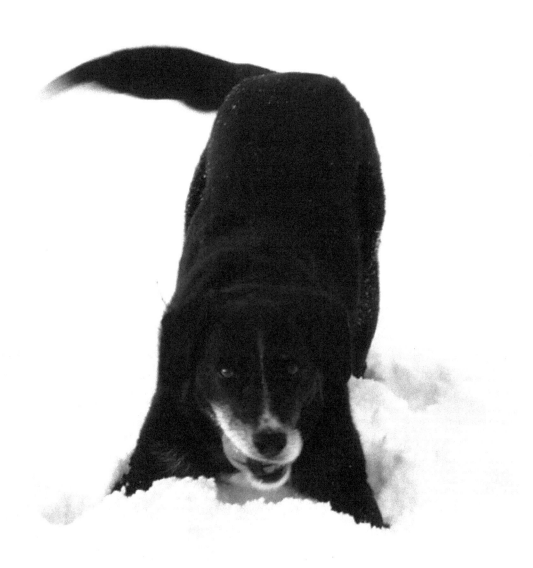

FOREWORD

By Nick Thompson, BSc (Vet Sci) Hons,
BVM&S, VetMFHom, MRCVS

Plants are medicinal, but why? Because they've been on the planet a lot longer than us mammals. If you think about it, plants were on the land and in the seas while we were evolving from bacteria and unicellular organisms into simple plankton-like creatures in the primordial oceans.

Over millennia, mammalian bodies developed and became incredibly complex, with 20,000 proteins, double helix DNA and complex phospho-lipid membranes, to name but a few of the wondrous structures that maintain life. Many thousands of biological chemicals are required within our bodies to keep this incredible mechanism ticking.

Animals first used plants as food. Food came with other life-giving chemicals, known as secondary metabolites, that the evolving creatures gradually adapted to utilise within their own bodies. Oceanic, and then terrestrial, plants became an external library of molecules that could help (or harm) the healthy functioning of a creature's metabolism. In this way, plants were the first medicines. With the advent of synthetic medicine, plant medicine fell from mainstream use. Now we are relearning to use plants and plant products to heal, alongside our modern diagnostics and the best of modern medicine.

Humans call plants that nourish 'vegetables', or 'grains', or 'fruit' and so on. They call plants that heal 'herbs'. Some of the active ingredients in plants and herbs are the secondary metabolites, the aromatic essential oils. Essential oils are concentrated, powerful elements of herbs and plants, which the mammalian body can recognise and use to help the delicate equilibrium we call health.

It is crucial that all those who work with aromatics to promote health and address disease are knowledgeable of the benefits and pitfalls in using each of these oils. This book represents a cornucopia of information and ideas to help furnish the concerned animal carer, the budding therapist, or holistic veterinarian with safe, practical and vital information.

I'm pleased to see Nayana has also explored stress. Humans in modern industrial societies are usually stressed. They are worried about money, or relationships, or the state of society, or all three and more! They create an internal environment in their bodies dominated by cortisone, the stress hormone, which gradually weakens tissue, breaks down organs and suppresses immune function. The result is chronic degenerative disease, cancer and depression; modern disease for modern people.

Unfortunately we do the same to our animals. They, too, show 'modern disease'. Our dogs and cats demonstrate more and more behavioural problems. Cats, dogs and horses express immune dysfunction as allergies and intolerances. In veterinary practice today, we see degenerative disease of joints, skin and organs manifesting in more and more exotic ways.

Self-selected aromatic essential oils, combined with an awareness of the supreme importance of stress on the mammalian body, together with a thorough knowledge of nutrition, give the intelligent animal guardian invaluable tools to promote health, heal disease, and maintain well-being.

INTRODUCTION

This book is a complete guide to using essential oils, hydrosols, vegetable and herbal oils (aromatic plant extracts) for animal health and well-being. The book contains useful information for every animal lover, whether a newcomer to the world of aromatics or an advanced student, guardian to one dog, or a veterinarian.

The book explains: how to use essential oils safely, which ones to use, and when; which essential oils are best for specific diseases; and how essential oils, hydrosols, herbal oils and a holistic attitude can benefit the animals in your care. Within these covers you will find the history of my personal experience with animals and essential oils, including stories and photographs of animals who have been helped by myself and my students.

As part of my holistic approach I use Traditional Chinese Medicine's Five Element Theory. The book explains how this can enhance your use of essential oils, give you a deeper understanding of your pet's character, and help you keep him healthy and happy.

Stress is one of the leading causes of health and behavioural problems, this book clarifies what stress really is, how to recognise it in animals and how to reduce mental and physical stress in your animal's environment.

Essential oils, herbal oils and hydrosols offer a unique, natural way of keeping our animals healthy and happy in a respectful and non-invasive way. The basics of how to use essential oils are easy to grasp, and this comprehensive guide will help you choose the right essential oil for every occasion, and explain how your animal can be an active participant in his own healing, self-selecting the remedies he feels he needs.

Aromatherapy could be considered one of the most 'scientific' of all the alternative medicine modalities because the properties of many essential oils have been researched for the food and beauty industries. The therapeutic potential of essential oil components has also been the subject of medical research since the last century. Simple medical trials with essential oils are not uncommon, among other things they are being investigated as a possible replacement for conventional drugs as antibiotic therapy starts to fail.

It is perfectly possible to use essential oils in the reductionist scientific fashion of "Oil X, at dosage Y, will cure disease Z. However, my experience with animals has shown me that healing is a natural art as much as it is a science and we cannot always explain how essential oils work through the prism of science. Essential oils work at an emotional and energetic level, which may be why inhaling miniscule amounts of essential oil can cause physical problems to resolve. My great wish is that through the way animals interact with essential oils, humans can learn to trust a more subtle approach to healing and the innate wisdom of all animals, including the human variety.

Animals love interacting with aromatics, and with the help of this book you can be certain you are giving your companions the essential oils they need to he healthy and happy, in a safe, effective way.

HOW TO USE THIS BOOK

This book is both an instruction manual and a reference resource, designed as an easy-to-use practical guide to using aromatic extracts for animal well-being.

The first part of the book provides you with a thorough understanding of why, how, and when to use essential oils; plus all the information you need to use essential oils and hydrosols safely and effectively. I suggest you read through everything before starting to use the oils on your animals, especially **Chapter 2, "How to use essential oils with animals"**.

Once you understand how and why to use the essential oils, you can use the book as a reference any time you want to find the best essential oil for your animal.

All the information you need in order to choose the right oil for every situation is in the **Materia Aromatica, (MA)** on pages 91 -230. Just follow these simple steps:

- Find the condition, or problem that you want to treat in **MA2**, Essential Oils and Hydrosols For Specific Conditions, on pages 98-108. Essential oils to help that condition are listed here. Cross reference these oils using **MA1**.

- **MA1** (Essential Oil & Hydrosol Cross Reference Chart), on pages 92-97 will show you which of the oils from the **MA2** listing best match your animal's problem, history, and character. Make a shortlist of a few likely oils.

- To learn more about the essential oils you have chosen and how they can help, read the individual profile in **MA3**, Essential Oil Profiles, on pages 109-206.

- Follow the instructions in Chapter 2, on how to help your animal select the essential oil he needs.

Alternatively you could start by checking **MA6**, Therapeutic Actions of Essential Oils on page 226, and select an essential oil by its action, e.g. anti-inflammatory, calming, sedative, etc. Continue with Steps 2 and 3 as normal.

To make flea spray, or other common topical remedies, go to **Chapter 5, How to Make Natural Lotions & Potions**. Here you will find instructions and recipes for making 100% natural skincare products for horses, dogs and cats.

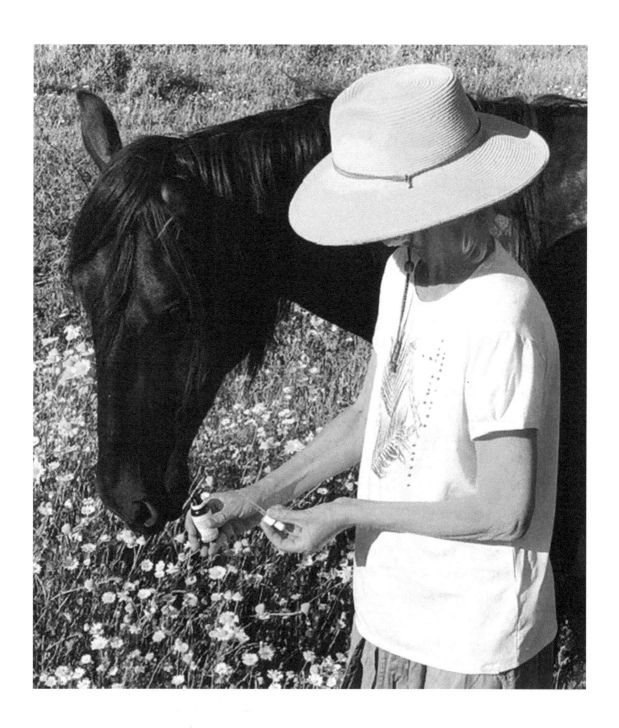

PROLOGUE

—

AMAZING AROMATICS

How it all started

Animals have always been a central part of my life. One of my earliest memories is the smell of warm pony in an English summer, and a cat was my first best friend. Horses are my passion, dogs my playmates, cats my soul mates; any animal that others find problematic has always been especially attractive to me. It seems I was born with a knack for understanding animals and have always tried to help people and animals understand each other better.

Essential oils came into my life in 1997. I am not someone who believes in things easily, but the first time I saw an animal interact with an essential oil I was a convert. I was working with 'problem' horses and their people when I read an article about aromatherapy for animals. Shortly after, I was on my way to visit a horse who needed my help so I grabbed whatever essential oils I had to hand in my bathroom to experiment for myself.

The horse I was going to see had multiple problems, separation anxiety, fear of cows, dogs, and leaving his field, and when stabled he spun around and around his box endlessly, a stereotypical behaviour. I offered the horse Roman chamomile, *(Anthemis nobilis)*, a calming oil, holding the open bottle outside his stable door, and watched, amazed, as his frenzied pacing gradually slowed down, and he stood with his head over the door half asleep.

After three minutes of standing in a trance, the horse looked me in the eyes, breathed deeply, reached his nose out to me, and gave me his trust, something that can take weeks to build with a traumatised horse. This was the beginning of his healing journey and my learning adventure.

From that moment, I knew I had to explore the potential in these powerful little potions. I went on to study Animal Aromatherapy from Caroline Ingraham, who pioneered the method of allowing animals to self-select the essential oils they need, earning my certificate in Animal

Aromatherapy and Healing Touch for Animals in 1999. I intended simply to use the essential oils to support my work with problem horses, but small brown bottles of fragrant delight have infiltrated my life and my work and expanded my horizons beyond horses to include all animals.

I really don't know how anyone lives without essential oils, especially if you have animals in your care (and that includes the human animal). I can't count the number of times I reach for my essential oils in a day, helping my animals stay healthy and happy, but here is an example of a typical day.

A day in the life of essential oils

As I fix myself a cup of tea at 6 a.m. after feeding the horses, I notice Gipsy, my old (mature!) dog is bugging me for something in her own polite way, shadowing me, staring, and sometimes pushing into me gently. This is un-usual behaviour for my self-contained Water dog and can mean only one thing: she needs oils.

Gipsy has been one of my primary tutors in the use of essential oils and the art of listening. The first time I offered her oils, when I had just started studying, she ran from me in horror and it took her quite a while not to disappear every time she saw a little brown bottle. This taught me not to offer dogs undiluted essential oils ini-tially, as it can be too overwhelming. It turns out that Gipsy is very sensitive to the oils so tiny amounts trigger big changes, but nowadays she lets me know when she needs them .

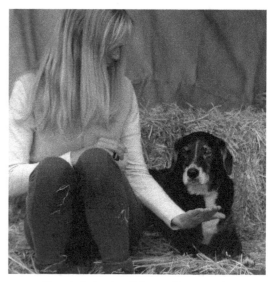

Gipsy inhales the oil I am offering with a dreamy look in her eye.

Gipsy's ability to communicate what she needs is highly refined and she leads my hands to her ear, which is bleeding from a small tear on the outer edge. Out comes **oregano** hydrosol *(Origanum vulgare)*, a teaspoon in a bowl of warm water and I wash the area liberally. Gipsy agrees and does not move away, wriggle or otherwise object. Then, to stop the bleeding, ease the pain, and protect from infection, I mix one drop each of **yarrow** *(Achillea millefolium)* and **lavender** *(Lavandula officinalis)* essential oil in a tablespoon of aloe vera gel and dollop some of that on. Gipsy says thank you and goes to lie down.

Next, I go down to the barn; the flies are bad already so I make a batch of fly spray. The three year old stallion, fresh in from the hills, is not sure about domestic life and things like fly spray, so I let him choose which essential oils and hydrosol go in the spray today, which will help him accept and enjoy the experience of being sprayed, instead of tensing up and scooting away.

I let the stallion smell various essential oils and hydrosols to see which ones he likes, he chooses **cedarwood** *(Cedrus Atlantica)*, calming and strengthening in times of change, **ylang-ylang** *(Cananga odorata)*, euphoric and relaxing, and *(Oreganum majorana)*, relaxing and anaphrodisiac (reduces sex-drive). I mix these oils into **neem** oil *(Azidirachta Indica)*, a brilliant natural pesticide, and let him lick a little of the mixture from my hands. I then add the hydrosol he liked, **lemongrass** *(Cymbopogon citratus)*, a dash of vinegar to help the oil and water mix, shake well, and spray. After an initial startle at the sound of the sprayer my 'wild' stallion stands relaxed, head low, ears half-cocked as I give him a good spray all over. Then he nuzzles my hand at the end. The first training session is over for the day.

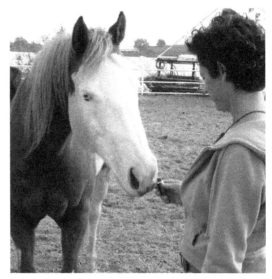

Bonita chooses rosemary essential oil for her circulation

I then dilute the mixture further with distilled water and give the dogs a good soaking as well, to keep them free of fleas and ticks. Lia, the beautiful, white, three-year old saluki cross, is even more sensitive than Gipsy to the strong fragrances, but when she needs help keeping flea-free, she allows me to spray her, and shows me exactly which spots would be most helpful (usually on her tummy and around her ears).

Next: is Bonita limping? Maybe, slightly. Bonita, a 15-year-old Paint mare, suffers from navicular, a degenerative disease of the foot bone, and often needs help from essential oils to keep the circulation flowing strongly. I offer her **plai** *(Zingiber cassumunar)* and **rosemary** *(Rosmarinus officinalis)* to smell. She chooses the rosemary, a heating, circulation stimulant, but is not to interested in the plai, a cooling anti-inflammatory, so I conclude that she is not suffering from pain, but appreciates the stimulant powers of rosemary to keep her going. I offer to rub some rosemary on the leg as well, but she just wants to sniff the bottle. I pass through all the older horses to see if anyone needs anything for aches and pains, but everyone seems happy this morning.

Then a livery owner arrives to ride with her Jack Russell puppy in tow. The pup will have to stay shut in the office while she is out, to keep him safe. He does not appreciate our concern for his safety and starts whining to be released. I add five drops of neroli *(Citrus aurantium)* hydrosol to a saucer of water, and put it down beside his drinking water. When we close the door again, the puppy whines a few times then turns to the bowl of neroli (which steadies the nerves and strengthens the heart, especially when missing someone), takes a few little licks and curls up beside it to doze until his person returns an hour later.

Now it's Ayla's turn. A three-year-old quarter horse filly, here for training, she has spent most of her life standing in a corral, eating and being told she is oh-so-cute, so is finding the whole concept of learning rather stressful. She is expressing this stress by obsessing about food and refusing to pick up any of my overtures to connect in movement. I want to encourage her to engage her brain and discover the fun we can have when playing together. I also think she is carrying a trauma from the accident she had at three months old, which has made her shut down awareness of the right side of her face. She almost lost her eye when she was hit in the face by a splintered plank (an unfortunate mishap, not abuse) and when I ask her to do something from that side, it is as if I am not there. It is quite common for animals to shut down an area of their body after traumatic injury.

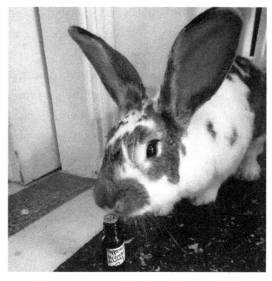

You can use essential oils with any animal once you understand the basic principal of animal self-selection.

I offer Ayla **angelica root** *(Angelica archangelica)*, for early childhood trauma and a feeling of grounded protection, yarrow to release trauma, rosemary to stimulate the brain and help her concentrate, and **lemon** *(Citrus limonum)*, for a clear mind and a sense of playful trust. She has a good sniff of the angelica, gets into a deep trance with the yarrow, refuses the rosemary and licks lemon from my hand. Later in the day we have a really good 'training' session and she manages to take instructions from the right side.

Next, I get a call from our local horse vet. Do I have a good solution for an allergy to fly bites as she would rather not give steroids? Do I? Of course! **Basil** *(Ocimum basilicum)* and great mugwort *(Artemesia arborescens)* melt away itchy, reactive bites, including bee and wasp stings, so I go up to the house to make up a batch.

At the house, I am met by big, black Goosh, the oversized Labrador-cross, wagging his tail forlornly and flapping his ear. What? Not another wounded dog! Goosh's left ear is black and gunky. Now I know it is Late Summer and Goosh's tendency to Damp Heat has got on top of him, which is the Chinese Medical way of saying he has a fungal infection in his ear. I need a cool, drying, anti-fungal oil to help him, and will take extra care that he doesn't get any junk food (anything other than fresh meat and veg). This is tough on a Labrador, but it's tough love that works.

Goosh chooses **myrrh** *(Commiphora myrrha)* essential oil, diluted in **calendula** macerated oil. He licks it off my hand enthusiastically and I wipe his ear out with it. Later, I will wash the ear with oregano and lavender hydrosol as well, but now it's lunchtime. In the afternoon, I go on to check whether any of the horses who have a tendency to itch need any essential oils to smell, or lotions applied; dress a nasty scrape on a horse's back leg with **garlic** *(Allium sativum)* essential oil in shea butter (antibiotic, skin repairant and keeps the flies off), and reach for the Traumagon, my own "first aid in a bottle", when my foot finds itself stuck under a horses hoof. Just one day in the life of an animal aromaticist.

I have been using essential oils to help animals and their guardians live healthier, happier lives since 1997. I have had the honour of working with a wide range of species: ferrets, rabbits, cats, dogs, horses, cows, sheep, goats, chickens, parrots, llamas, monkeys and, yes, even the occasional human. I still get a thrill every time I see how much animals enjoy interacting with essential oils, and great satisfaction from being able to help them.

In this book I share with you my love and knowledge of aromatic extracts and how they can help you and your animals live healthy, happy lives, naturally.

"Odors have a power of persuasion stronger than that of words, appearances, emotions, or will. The persuasive power of an odor cannot be fended off, it enters into us like breath into our lungs, it fills us up, imbues us totally. There is no remedy for it."

- Patrick Süskind

CHAPTER 1

GETTING TO KNOW ESSENTIAL OILS

Background check

An essential oil is like any tool, the better you know how it works the more effectively you can use it. I always approach an essential oil as if getting to know a colleague, learning about its background and the environment that has created it, until I have a clear picture of its character and capabilities. This section will introduce you to essential oils, what they are and what they can do before going on to get intimate with the individual oils.

So what are essential oils?

One would think with the prevalence of essential oils in our shampoos today this would be an easy question to answer, but did you know that most essential oils are not even oily? To answer this question fully we need to look at essential oils from various angles.

BIOLOGICALLY SPEAKING

Explosive stuff

Essential oils are secondary plant metabolites, molecules produced as part of the plant's survival mechanism and stored within the plant until needed; almost every plant contains at least a small quantity of essential oil.

Essential oils are fragrant; the smell when you crush lavender, or peel an orange is the essential oil exploding into the air as it is released. Essential oils can be found in petals, roots, leaves, bark, or resin according to their function. In different plants they have different functions, some of which are assumed to be:

- » To prevent attack by insects and herbivores;
- » To protect against and fight off bacteria and fungi;
- » To attract insects to pollinate the plant;
- » To help heal wounds, e.g. oozing tree resins containing anti-bacterial components;
- » To prevent other plants growing near them; and,
- » To protect from dehydration by creating a haze of essential oil.

HISTORICALLY SPEAKING

Humans have valued aromatic healing substances for a long, long time. In pre-historic times, humans would still have been have been guided by an innate ability to know which herbs were helpful, as all animals are. As humans developed it is likely they also learned about the healing properties of plants by watching what animals ate.

Aromatics through the ages

Early History: Aromatic herbs have been used by humans for religious rituals & healing as far back as we know.

3,000 BC: First known still.

10th Century: Avicenna refined the art of distillation.

13th Century: Eastern aromatics popularised by returning Crusaders, distillation of local herbs begins.

16th Century: Essential oils and floral waters an accepted part of the medical pharmacopeia.

19th Century: Scientific analysis of essential oil components begins, leading to development of some our most common synthetic medicines.

20th Century: Popularisation of essential oils in beauty therapy and holistic massage.

1980s: Caroline Ingraham starts to develop the use of essential oils for animal health using the principle of self-selection.

Till present: Continuing research in and development of aromatic extracts for animal well-being.

There are many references to aromatic substances in early religious and medical literature, although it is unclear if this was the distilled essential oil, or the burning of aromatic gums, resins and herbs. The earliest known distillation equipment was discovered in Pakistan and dates from 3000 b.c.

Early written history

The earliest written references to the use of incense and unguents in spiritual and healing ceremonies (in those days, often one and the same) all come from around 2000 b.c. when we have the first written 'medical texts' from India, China and Egypt.

The Old Testament also refers to aromatics, such as the 'Holy herb' hyssop, a symbol of spiritual cleansing. The fact that myrrh and frankincense were gifts fit for a king also tells us something about the cultural importance of aromatics.

Essential oils and herbal healing

The ancient knowledge of herbal healing, which included aromatics, was passed down through the Greeks, the Romans, and the Arabs, each great civilisation inheriting the wisdom from the previous one and building on the body of knowledge. It was Avicenna, a great scientist of the 10th century, who is credited with improving and refining the art of distillation to extract pure essential oil from the aromatic water.

Perfumes of Arabia

By the 13th century, aromatics, 'the perfumes of Arabia', arrived in Europe with the returning Crusaders, as Europe awoke from its Dark Age; rose water was always a favourite. People also began to scatter aromatic herbs and bouquets through the straw-lined floors of their houses, to ward off disease and keep away fleas. As the use of aromatics became a part of everyday life, people started to distil local plants and herbs such as peppermint, sage and lavender. These were considerably less expensive than exotic foreign oils and resins, and widely available.

By the 16th century, distilled oils and aromatic water were an accepted part of the medic's tool kit and people started to record the uses and properties of essential oils. And it is said that the distillation of plant matter into volatile substances inspired the alchemists to try to distil gold from base metal.

In the 19th century, it became possible to analyse essential oils scientifically, breaking them down into their constituent parts, trying to find out what made them work. This led to the development of synthetic fragrance and modern synthetic medicine, which, ironically, led to the devaluation of essential oils to perfumery and flavouring substances. The healing powers of essential oils and aromatic waters may have been lost to us if it hadn't been for the actions of a careless chemist.

The careless chemist

In 1920 the French chemist Rene-Maurice Gattefosse was researching the cosmetic properties of essential oils in his family's laboratory when he burned his hand severely. Lacking anything else convenient (so the story goes), he plunged his hand into a vat of lavender essential oil and his pain was immediately relieved; the wound also healed without infection or scarring. This led him to focus his research on the medicinal properties of essential oils and to coin the term *aromatherapie*.

Lovely lavender!

Lavender is one of the best loved and most widely used essential oils. I think it fitting that common lavender triggered the popularity of essential oils today, all because of the speed with which it healed a careless chemist's burnt hand.

It is easy to be snooty about this widely used and sometimes highly adulterated oil, but a good quality Lavender essential oil has a huge range of actions.

If I was allowed only one essential oil, I would sigh a little about leaving better loved and more sophisticated essential oils at home, but I would have to pack my lavender.

Another Frenchman, Dr Jean Valnet started to study the medical uses of essential oils when he was caring for soldiers in World War II. Due to a shortage of supplies, Dr Valnet used essential oils to heal wounds and infections. He also used them successfully in the care of psychiatric patients. In France and Germany, physicians trained in aromatic medicine still prescribe essential oils internally, by mouth or via rectal or vaginal pessaries.

Madame Maury, also French, developed the use of massage as a delivery of essential oils, as a result of her research on the effects of essential oils on the skin and musculature. During the 1960s/1970s, aromatherapy massage was established in the UK as a healing modality by the likes of Robert and Maggie Tisserand, Shirley Price and Patricia Davies. Nowadays many people in the medical care business, especially in Europe recognise how essential oils can help relieve symptoms and reduce stress for patients.

Animal aromatherapy

In the 1980's, Caroline Ingraham studied aromatherapy and kinesiology with Robert Tisserand. Soon after qualifying as an aromatherapist she started to experiment with using essential oils on her own pets and had some dramatic results. Because of these successes, with the help of interested vets, Caroline started to explore the use of essential oils with animals more fully.

During this time, Caroline started to notice that animals would show a definite preference for one essential oil over another. Depending on their life experience and present problems, and they would clearly indicate which oils they wanted.

From this observation, supported by research in the developing science of zoopharmacognosy (the study of animal self-medication in the wild), Caroline developed the method of allowing animals to select their essential oils and guide their own healing. In 1995, Caroline started to teach others and animal aromatherapy became more widely known.

Although essential oils have a tradition of use in veterinary medicine, this modern style of essential oil therapy for animals is a young

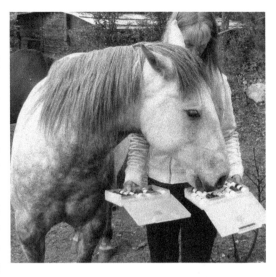

Animals are able to choose the exact essential oil they want/need from among the 60 bottles in my case. Here, Shanti indicates what she wants by nibbling at a bottle.

discipline and developing all the time. Using self-selection as our guide has proved to be safe and effective, and easy to teach to animal guardians, so you can confidently include aromatic extracts in your home pharmacy.

CHEMICALLY SPEAKING

A basic understanding of the chemical make-up of essential oils can help your overall understanding of how they work, even if you are one of the many 'chemistry phobics', don't skip this section. The information is simple but powerful.

Functional members of a group

Essential oils are made up of relatively simple compounds combining mainly carbon, hydrogen and oxygen to produce at least 3,000 different aromatic molecules. Each molecule belongs to a specific functional group according to its basic structure and these groups can be expected to have similar actions.

For example: **aldehydes** are anti-infectious, analgesic and anti-inflammatory; **esters** are calming, sedative, anti-spasmodic and mucolytic; **alcohols and phenols** are anti-pathogenic and immune stimulant.

Essential oils contain molecules from a variety of functional groups. Most essential oils have between 20 and 50 easily identifiable components but can have up to 200. Each oil's unique combination of components creates its aroma, its therapeutic effect, and how safe it is to use.

Everybody counts!

Each component is as significant to the overall efficacy of the oil as the major parts. For example a study done on Cymbopogon citratus (DC.) Stapf., commonly known as lemon grass found that while the alpha-citral (geranial) and beta-citral (neral) components individually elicit antibacterial action on gram-negative and gram-positive organisms, myrcene enhanced the activities when mixed with either of the other two main components , even though alone it had little or no effect. (Onawunmi, GO, Yisak WA, Ogunlana EO. (1984). Antibacterial constituents in the essential oil of Cymbopogon citratus. J. Ethnopharmacol. Dec;12(3):279-86.)

United we stand!

Whole essential oil is often safer than isolated components as well, because the whole oil often contains small amounts of a chemical that can neutralise the effect of potentially damaging chemicals. For example, the aldehyde citral can cause a chemical burn when applied to skin, but if you add 20% d-limonene to the citral it becomes harmless. Most citral rich essential oils naturally contain sufficient d-limonene to render the citral harmless. Nature's system of checks and balances is quite mind-boggling and means that the whole oil is nearly always safer and more effective than any of the component parts. This synergy of constituents is also what makes synthetic imitations inferior.

Location, location!

The chemical make-up of essential oil is affected by various factors, from where and how the plant is grown, to how it is harvested, distilled and stored. For instance, lavender grown above 1000 metres is chemically different to that grown at lower altitudes. The chemical content of the earth, and how much sunshine a plant receives also affect the final makeup. The variation in chemical make-up of plants is called a chemotype (ct) and affects both the fragrance of an essential oil and its therapeutic actions.

ENERGETICALLY SPEAKING

Aromatic substances have been connected with spiritual practice from the earliest recorded history at the least, and the symbolism of fragrant smoke rising to the heavens carrying messages to the gods seems obvious and right. Fragrance has a powerful effect on the human psyche and can create moods and feelings that must have looked magical to more innocent people than we. Sages and visionaries from all traditions have used aromatics to help them connect to the spirit world, seeking answers beyond themselves.

Alchemists were inspired to try to make base metal into gold after seeing how essential oils could be distilled from plant matter, which they saw as an analogy for turning gross matter (Man) into spirit, or the refining of energy. Essential oils have played a role in the meditative traditions as well as an energetic support to uplift the spirits, and keep the spirit connected to the body.

The etheric nature of essential oils, their lightness of touch, makes them powerful energetic agents that can interact with the mammalian bio-system at multiple levels, healing and inspiring, on a mental, emotional and energetic level, as well as physically.

Functional groups commonly found in essential oils, and their actions

Monoterpenes: present in most essential oils, antiseptic, analgesic (minimal), skin disinfectant, fortifying, cortisone like. Can be aggressive to skin and mucous membranes. Name ends in ene, e.g. limonene, pinene.

Sesquiterpenes: antiseptic, hypotensive, bactericidal, calming, anti-tumour. e.g chamazulene, -bisabolene.

Monoterpenols: anti-infective, anti-bacterial, antiviral, stimulant, non-irritant. Name ends in 'ol', e.g. linalol, geraniol.

Sesquiterpenols: similar to above but also venous & lymphatic decongestants. Name ends in end 'ol', e.g. farnesol, cedrol.

Phenols: very powerful compounds, antiseptic, bactericidal, immune & nervous stimulant, can be toxic to liver and irritant to skin, keep away from cats, carvacrol, eugenol, thymol.

Aldehyde: calming, hypotensive, antiviral, analgesic, anti-inflammatory, febrfuge. Possible skin irritant. Name ends in 'al', e.g. neral, geranial, citronellal.

Ketones: related to above, not often found in essential oils but are significant. Calming, sedative, cicatrisant, mucolytic, lipolytic, analgesic, anti-coagulant, expectorant, digestive. Can be neurotoxic or abortifacient, use with caution. Name ends in 'one', e.g. verbenone, menthone. Do not use essential oils containing thujone or pugelone.

Acids and esters: antifungal, anti-inflammatory, antispasmodic, calming, e.g. linalyl acetate.

PERSONALLY SPEAKING

Essential oils interact with each individual on a very personal level; your character and health issues will affect how you experience each essential oil. Ultimately the best way to get to know an essential oil is to use it on yourself. First of all smell the oil (I find this irresistible!). It is important that you smell the oil with awareness, which means be conscious of your responses and which parts of the body the oil stimulates; smell it with each side of your nostril like animals do. Some essential oils you will love and return to again and again, others you will like only when you need them, some you will always dislike but will grow to respect. By using essential oils on yourself, knowledge goes beyond theory and becomes part of your being, and you start to understand them intuitively.

Getting to know an essential oil

Choose an essential oil you like, or think you need, open the bottle, smell it with each nostril and ask yourself:

- » How does it make me feel?
- » Which part of my body does it affect?
- » What temperature is it?
- » What colour does it invoke?
- » Is the impact the same with each nostril?
- » Does the oil affect me differently if diluted?

Put a drop of oil on a tissue or blotting paper and smell it at hourly intervals, note how the smell changes as the oil dries out. Keep the oil with you all day, smell it at different times and in different moods and note how you feel about it each time. Put a few drops of diluted oil in your bath, or dilute it and dab it on your wrists, in other words, explore it thoroughly.

HOW DO ESSENTIAL OILS AFFECT HEALTH?

Physically

Essential oils are highly volatile, which means they evaporate and disperse as soon as they are exposed to the air. In effect, this means they are exploding out of the bottle and up into our olfactory system when we take the lid off a bottle. When we breathe, the molecules are absorbed into the moist lining of the nose, from where they pass quickly into the blood, and brain, and affect the nervous system.

The olfactory area of the brain (the one that receives and processes smells) lies within the limbic system, one of the earliest parts of the brain to evolve. The limbic system is concerned with instincts, mood, emotions, and memory. These can be transformed into physical responses through the hypothalamus, via the autonomic nervous system.

Odour stimuli (smells), cause neurotransmitters such as endorphins, serotonin and noradrenalin to be released in the limbic system. Depending on their range of influence, neurotransmitters can help reduce pain, relax the mind or body, calm, stimulate, sedate, awaken and create feelings of well-being. In addition, the limbic system also affects emotional aspects of behaviour: pain, pleasure, anger, fear, sorrow, and affection. Sexuality can be released, heightened, or subdued through the release of hormones in the endocrine system.

Because essential oil molecules are very small, they pass easily through the skin when applied topically and enter the bloodstream. This is the most common form of delivery for humans.

Animals generally prefer to lick or sniff the oils and dramatic results can be seen without any topical application. Although animals lick the oils, it is my belief that this is an enhanced method of inhaling (taste and smell being almost the same function). The amount of essential oil that goes into the digestive system when an animal licks is negligible as most of it is absorbed into the mucous membranes. A large part of it is excreted through the lungs after inhalation; any that enters the blood system will pass through the liver and be excreted through the kidneys,

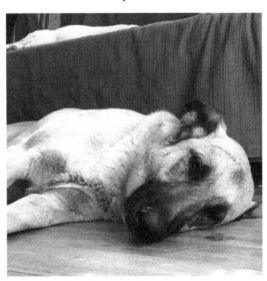

This dog may look like he's taking a nap, but if you look closely you can see his eyes are open and he is in a trance after inhaling essential oil.

Psychologically

Because essential oils interact with the limbic system, they have a direct influence on the neurotransmitters that control emotion, so they affect mental/emotional states.

One of aromatherapy's great benefits is stress reduction. This is due not only to the effect of the essential oils, but also because animals are being offered a choice. All too often, out of our care and concern for their welfare, our animals are denied choice of any kind.

This loss of control is stressful in its own right. By giving the animal the opportunity to select what it needs to help it feel better (as it would in nature), we relieve that stress. This affects the psyche profoundly, allowing the animal to drop behaviours that have developed from living in a constant state of low-grade stress.

Energetically

For some people the concept of energy is hard to understand; seeing is believing and for most people energy is something that is felt rather than seen. Kirlian photography is a technique of high-frequency photography that displays the patterns and colours of the body's energy or auric field, making energy fields visible. Kirlian photography was used to photograph a human hand before and after the application of a drop of essential oil. After the essential oil was applied the colourful pattern around the hand, known as the aura, increased in size and colour. This suggests that essential oils heighten the healing power of touch by increasing the electrical charge. Each essential oil also has a specific aura when photographed, proving they are energetically charged.

How essential oils work

1. Essential oils evaporate when exposed to air.
2. The fragrance is inhaled.
3. Tiny essential oil molecules pass through the nose lining into the blood and brain.
4. Essential oils enter the limbic system of the brain affecting emotions and relaxation response.
5. The hypothalamus converts the brain stimuli into physical functions, such as decreased heartbeat, anti-inflammatory response, etc.

When the body (or the universe!) is viewed holistically it can be seen as a mass of electrically charged, pulsating molecules that group together to make one form visible. When something interrupts the flow of electricity within a bio-mass, such as an accident, emotional trauma or stress of any kind, the circuit breaks and eventually that part of the system will run out of energy. This will manifest as an imbalance in the body or mind, what we call illness or behaviour problems.

Energetically and physically, I see essential oils as the messengers of the universe: the fragrance of the rose attracts insects, the fragrance of eucalyptus repels them. Essential oils continue this role when they interact with a body system, sending out electrical/energetic messages to reconnect circuits that are broken. Possibly this is why you can see animals change their behaviour after inhaling the appropriate essential oil just once.

HOW ARE ESSENTIAL OILS PRODUCED?

Steam distillation

Essential oils are extracted from fresh or dry plant matter, usually by steam distillation. Pressurised steam is passed through the plant matter, the steam evaporates, the water is collected and the oils are separated from the water. The water that remains is known as hydrosol, hydrolat, or aromatic water, and is also used in aromatherapy. The temperature, pressure and length of time of the distillation affects the quality of the finished product; too much heat or pressure will destroy some of the molecules in the essential oil. Also, there is an optimum time for the distillation of each essential oil, as they can produce quite different qualities of oil as time proceeds, for example, the oil of ylang-ylang (Cananga odorata) is collected every hour through the distillation and sold accordingly (ylang-ylang extra is the product of the first hour, ylang-ylang 1 is the product of the 2nd hour etc.).

Cold pressing

Essential oil is extracted from citrus fruit peel by cold pressing; the skins are literally squeezed between two weights until all the essential oil is collected. No heat is used in this process which is good for the quality of the oil, but there is more chance for pesticides to pass over into the oil, so it is much more important to buy organic citrus peel oils.

Solvent extraction

Some raw materials are either too delicate (jasmine) or too inert (seaweed) to be steam-distilled and only yield their essential oil through other methods, such as solvent extraction or lipid absorption. This process uses a non-polar solvent, such as hexane, to separate oils from the plant matter, this is known as a concrete. The concrete is then washed with ethyl alcohol. After cooling, filtering and evaporation of the solvent, a wax-free oily residue remains, which is known as an absolute.

This method is costly and time-consuming and the final product, called an absolute, is sometimes contaminated by very low levels of solvent. For this reason, it is preferable to use steam-distilled or cold-pressed essential oils. However, there are some very useful oils, such as seaweed and jasmine, that are only available as absolutes, and I could not do without them. I just make sure when purchasing these oils that they are free of contaminants, by requesting a GC/MS from my supplier.

Ancient art

Extracting essential oil by enfleurage is an ancient art, originally developed by perfumers, especially in the Grasse region of France.

Nowadays enfleurage is considered inefficient and costly, but is still commonly used to extract essential oils from delicate floral botanicals such as jasmine and tuberose, which would be destroyed by the high temperatures of steam distillation.

These days, supercritical fluid extraction using liquid carbon dioxide (CO_2) or similar compressed gases is starting to replace the old-fashioned method.

CO2 extraction

Finally, there is a fairly new method of extraction known as CO_2 extraction, whereby carbon dioxide is subjected to pressure high enough to liquefy the gas. This liquid CO_2 can be used as an inert safe, liquid solvent in a process similar to that used to extract absolutes. The advantage is that no solvent residue remains as the CO_2 simply reverts to a gas and evaporates at normal pressure. Another advantage of this method is that plant matter is not heated so does not degrade.

A WORD ON QUALITY

Therapeutic vs industrial

Before we move on from the basics of what an essential oil is, a word on quality. Not all essential oils are created equal. The vast bulk of essential oils in the world are produced for the fragrance and flavouring industries, whose main concern is to get as much product for as little cost as possible. Essential oils produced in this way are not suitable for therapeutic use, as many of the more volatile components are destroyed in the distillation.

The difference between an oil of therapeutic quality and one produced for food flavouring is the difference between vintage wine and a grape soda. Therapeutic quality essential oils are distilled with care, which means slowly, over a lower heat.

Careful cultivation

The method of production also affects the quality and energy of an essential oil. The best oils come from single crop farmers who grow ethically, preferably organically and are involved with the essential oil from seeding through distillation. (Note: It is not always possible to find good quality certified organic essential oils due to the costs involved in certifying them.) Wild crafting (picking plants from the wild) sounds romantic but does not guarantee quality if the plant is harvested at the wrong time or without due care. If wild-crafting is undertaken without knowledge and respect for the plant it can be damaging to the environment. Over-harvesting has the potential to destroy a species if the plant does not have time to regenerate. It is very important that distillers can verify that wild plants are harvested ethically and with due care.

Purity

Many essential oils are adulterated, usually by the addition of synthetic fragrance or a cheaper essential oil with a similar fragrance. This is especially true of the more expensive oils such as rose or those in high demand, like French lavender.

The best way to guarantee you are using good quality oils is to buy from a reputable supplier of essential oils intended for therapeutic use, who can guarantee botanical purity, tell you where the plant was grown, and how it was distilled. Small companies whose clientele is primarily therapists generally carry the highest quality oils. Companies I recommend are listed at the end of the book.

Adultery is a dirty game!

An adulterated essential oil is one that has been tampered with, usually by:

» Blending less expensive essential oils with a more costly oil,

» Blending a higher quality essential oil with a lower grade version of the same species,

» Adding individual constituents, either natural or synthetic, to an essential oil, commonly linalyl acetate to lavender,

» Adding synthetics to improve the aroma, or,

» Adding vegetable oil.

The final judge

The more you educate your nose, the easier it will be for you to recognise a good quality essential oil. Every true essential oil is penetrative, exploding up your nose as you inhale. There is a medicinal edge to even the most floral of essential oils, and a complexity of fragrance that changes the longer you smell the oil.

The more essential oils you smell, the better you become at identifying all the individual fragrances they contain. Your nose will start to pick up notes that suggest the essential oil is adulterated, such as a scent that does not blend in harmoniously, or if the fragrance is too flat or too sweet. This is a skill that is easily learned, and pleasant too, so expose your nose to essential oils.

Keep it cool!

To ensure you maintain the quality of your essential oils, always store them in a cool, dark place with the lids tightly closed to minimise oxidisation. All essential oils sold in the EU (European Union) must have a two-year 'sell-by' date on the bottle, but many oils, especially the heavy, resinous ones such as patchouli, last for years, and some improve with age. Citrus and pine oils only last a year.

To review

Essential oils are volatile extracts of chemically bio-active plants that interact with the mammalian brain to activate biochemical responses, which trigger healing.

Factors in essential oil quality

» Quality of the soil,

» The weather,

» Organic or pesticide free cultivation of plants,

» How and when plant material is harvested,

» Storage of plant material prior to distillation,

» The type and material of distillation equipment,

» Temperature and pressure of distillation,

» Adulteration, standardisation or adjustments of the essential oil,

» Proper storage of essential oil from production until final use.

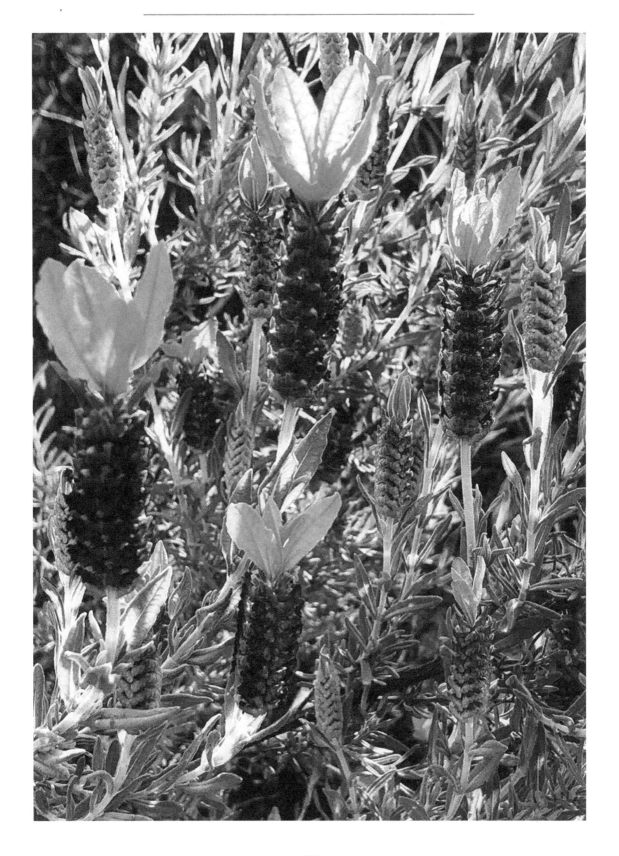

"Watch any plant or animal and let it teach you acceptance of what is, surrender to the Now. Let it teach you Being. Let it teach you integrity--which means to be one, to be yourself, to be real. Let it teach you how to live and how to die, and how not to make living and dying into a problem."

- Eckhart Tolle

CHAPTER 2

HOW TO USE ESSENTIAL OILS WITH ANIMALS

Self-selection: the first principle

The use of essential oils for animals is founded on the principle that animals know instinctively what they need for the maintenance of health. Animals have an innate ability to self-medicate. When left to their own devices they pick and choose the herbs they need to maintain health, and balance their diet to provide the nutrients they need.

I am always asked if domestic animals still have this instinct: indeed they do! In evolutionary terms the period of domestication is miniscule, certainly not enough time for significant changes in instinctual behaviour. Anyone who has a dog or cat will have seen them eat grass, dig up the houseplants, or drink from the muddiest puddle when they have good clean water at home. These are all forms of self-medication, as is eating dirt. Horses snatching at hawthorn or willow or similar as you ride by are also trying to get the medicine they need.

The feel-good factor

An animal's ability to pick what he needs is instinctive rather than acquired knowledge and is based on the 'hedonic' response. Hedonic feedback assumes that the animal perceives something as tasty according to bodily requirements. If it makes them feel good it must be good for them, so they will seek out those plants. Every animal tries to maintain homeostasis (the healthy functioning of a body system) and will take measures to return the system to balance when it is does not feel good.

One man's poison...

In her fascinating book *"Wild Health"*, Cindy Engel explains that animals are considered to be self-medicating when they eat plants not normally included in their diet. Often these are plants considered to be poisonous, but many substances that contain toxins are also antibacterial, anti-tumour, anti-inflammatory or otherwise medicinal. For example, Cindy cites that plants of the Senecio family, such as ragwort, considred to toxic to horses and cattle, causing liver damage when eaten often, can reduce cancerous tumours when eaten in small quantities.

Animals who have freedom to roam also have access to substances that can counteract the potentially toxic effects of healing plants. Eating clay or dirt is one way that animals counteract poison in the body. Wild animals will travel many miles to eat clay. Charcoal absorbs toxins in the stomach; moss and lichen are also anti-toxic, as are some plants. Animals also build tolerance to toxins by taking in a little at a time.

Case study 1 - Mathilda the Choosy Chicken

Early in my journey with essential oils, my partner jokingly asked if I could cure our broody hen, who would rather starve herself to death than leave the nest of eggs she had managed to gather. Mathilda was a tame and friendly hen so I tucked her under my arm and opened bottles of frankincense and rose. She cocked her head to one side then the other, and looked at me indulgently for a moment, then clearly went and pecked at the rose, looked at me and pecked again, then settled comfortably into my arms for a moment seeming to relax completely. After a couple of minutes she wriggled to get down and set to eating. I diluted a few drops of rose hydrosol in a saucer of water and left that for her as well. She pecked at the saucer and ate from the ground around it for a while then wandered off to her friends. From that day forth Mathilda's terrible drive to sit on eggs vanished completely.

Guided healing

From hens to humans, from rabbits to rhinos, we all know instinctively what is good for us. We must respect this when giving essential oils to animals. The ability to pick exactly what they need is so acute that I have watched dogs go through my collection of 60 essential oils, sniffing the closed bottles, to choose the oil they need. Every animal is clear about which essential oil it needs, how much and for how long, and if allowed they will guide us in their healing. Animals in our care rely on us to provide them with the means to self-medicate; essential oils give us the perfect way to fulfil this natural need, even if our animals never get closer to a wildflower meadow than the local park.

UNDERSTANDING RESPONSES

The art of listening

The art of successfully facilitating your animal's self-medication lies in interpreting your animal's reaction to the oil correctly. Above all, you need to be patient and observant. The good news is that every species I have worked with, from the mundane to the exotic, follows the same basic patterns of response, which makes interpreting the responses easy.

When you offer essential oils and hydrosols to your animal you must watch carefully, interpret her responses and follow her direction on how she wants to interact with the oils. This develops your listening and observational skills and makes you more attentive to your animal in all areas of your life.

The basic responses

When you first offer an oil for an animal to smell, they often look a little surprised or perplexed, sometimes even wary. If your animal likes the oil, he will then move closer, or keep his head turned towards you. If he does not like the oil, he will move away, put his head down, or otherwise avoid the smell.

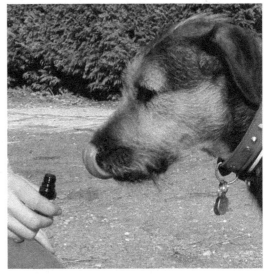

Animals always smell the oil with each nostril. This is easy to see with horses, who very deliberately move between the nostrils, the smaller the animal, the harder this is to detect, so watch carefully.

Licking the lips quickly is another indication of interest in the oil, particularly in carnivores. Cats and small animals often take just a small sniff, then a quick lick of their lips, move to a

Jessie shows interest. Note the big 'yummy' lick of her tongue and her focussed attention.

comfortable distance and settle down with their nose in the direction of the bottle.

Dogs also lick, a bigger 'yum-yum' lick, not to be confused with a large yawning lick, which can indicate they are feeling a little stressed and may need you to move the oil further away.

Animals will establish how far they want to be from the bottle. This may cause them walk away from the bottle initially. This is often interpreted as a negative response, but as long as the animal stays in the room with you, with their nose in your direction, it should be counted as a positive response.

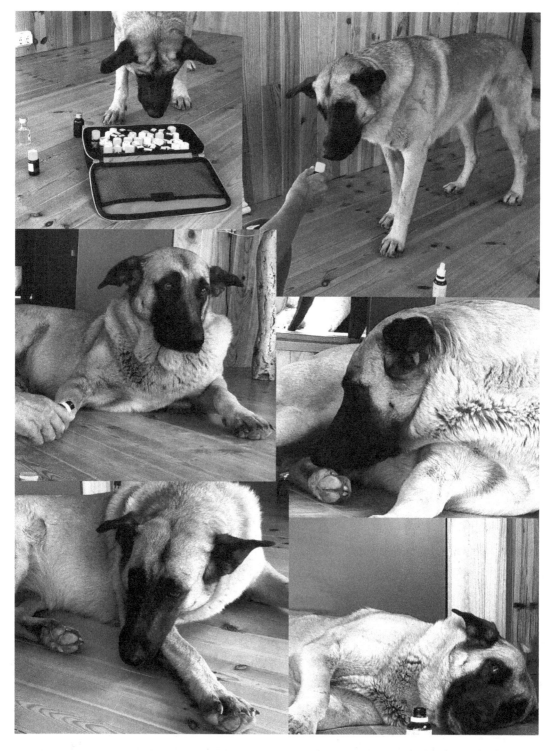

This is a typical sequence of a dog selecting an oil. First she picks from the box, then I verify her selection. She trances a little, then puts her nose to an acupressure point on her hind leg, then she puts her nose over her legs and finally, just lets herself go completely and lies flat out to process

It is important to allow the animal freedom of movement and to let him leave the area if he chooses. If you are not sure if an animal is just staying with you to be polite or really taking the oil in, check if his nostrils are twitching. If he is taking the oil you will see a slight flaring of the nostrils as he breathes in.

The individual response

Each species also has variations on the patterns of response, and the better you know the normal behaviour of the species, the easier it is to interpret what you are seeing. The most unique response I have ever had was from a bad-tempered llama, who spat at me when I offered an oil he didn't like, very unpleasant!

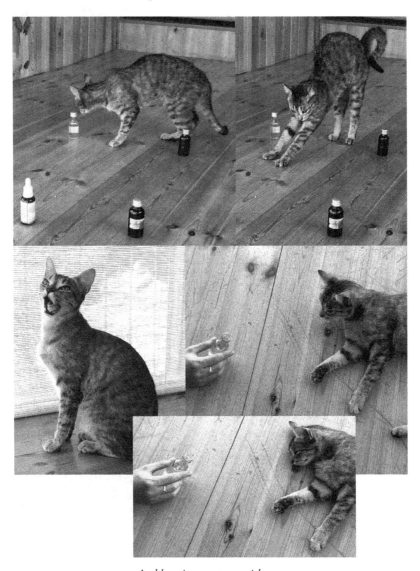

And here is a sequence with a cat

The character of each individual must also be taken into account. Give shy, withdrawn animals time to interact. Greedy, enthusiastic types need to have time to settle down and engage fully. A Labrador is likely to be demonstrative and forthright with the oils, probably wanting to lick them. A reserved greyhound may be more cagey about his responses, sniffing and then retreating, then coming back for another sniff, and so on.

Two extremes

Gipsy, a Labrador/collie/lurcher mix (and somewhat of a drama queen it has to be admitted!) usually lies down about two metres away from me to take in the oils, and looks very offended if I try to get any closer. As long as she has her body towards me and her nose is

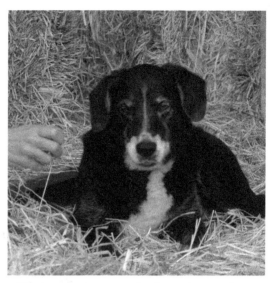

This is a strong response for Gipsy, she stays close to the bottle and wrinkles her nose.

twitching, I count it as a positive response. When she has finished, she will get up and walk away. On the other hand, my horse acts as if he likes every oil he is offered, but those he really needs he returns to and licks with his tongue, instead of just nibbling with his lips. If her really needs them, he goes into a trance, just inhaling.

THE THREE CATEGORIES OF RESPONSE

There are three major ways that an animal chooses to interact with aromatic extracts: smelling, licking, or localised topical application.

Inhalation

I consider inhalation the most powerful way to deliver essential oils, as they go straight into the brain via the olfactory system, altering the brain chemistry. The animal usually goes into a trance-like state, head lowered, eyes flickering as she processes the changes in her neurochemistry.

This trance can be the hardest response for the beginner to read, as it can appear the animal is just lying there doing nothing, or standing napping. If you observe carefully you will see the eyes flicker

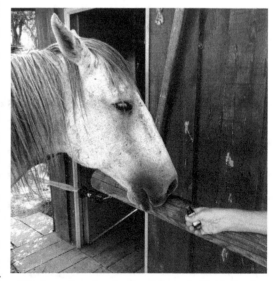

This horse breathes deeply with eyes half closed as he inhales the oil.

and nostrils flaring slightly. If you move the bottle away the animal will follow the aroma with her nose, or look at you. Once there is no reaction when you move the bottle, replace the lid and wait for your animal to return from his relaxed space before offering another oil. Do not hurry the process and do not try to offer other oils until she has 'come back'.

Oral

Animals are more likely to want the oils orally if they have a physical problem or one that is not very deeply rooted. The sense of smell and taste function together, and most essential oil taken into the mouth will be absorbed into the olfac-

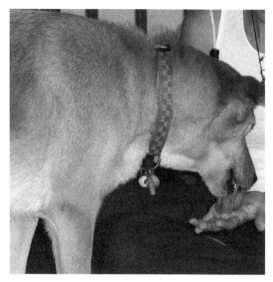

Nin licks diluted cedarwood oil enthusiastically

tory cavity. Some of the oil will be absorbed into the blood system via mucous membranes, but only a minimal amount will reach the digestive system. If your animal tries to lick the bottle or behaves very orally, dab a small amount of **diluted** oil on your hand, (or on a saucer or a bucket if they do not want to lick from your hand) and allow him to lick it off. Repeat this two or three times in a session.

While the animal is licking, keep the open bottle of oil in range of his nostrils so he is also inhaling the oil.

Topical

Occasionally, an animal may indicate that he wants the oil dabbed onto a particular spot, often an acupuncture point, by pointing with his head, stamping a foot, moving into you with his body or some unique method of communication all his own. In this case, just rub a little oil into the area he has indicated. *(Topical application may also be used for skin conditions, sprains and bruises; I explain how to make lotions and potions for that later.)*

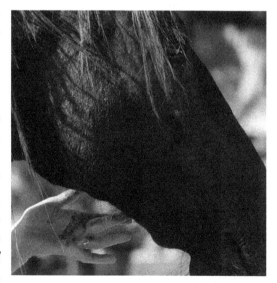

Leela rubbed her chin on me, so I gently ask if she wants topical application.

Move your hand into the area slowly, allowing the animal to move away if he does not want oil on his body after all, or guide you to the exact spot. Massage the area lightly until your animal moves away. Topical application is contraindicated for cats.

THREE LEVELS OF INTEREST

Initial interest

Animals are expected to be intensely interested in at least one essential oil at the beginning of a treatment, and usually they will show interest in two or three oils. Interest in each oil can vary from day to day; as treatment progresses your animal should lose interest in all the oils.

Normally animals will start to lose interest in the oils within three days to a week of the first session. In rare cases an animal will lose interest after one session, especially if the problem was not deep-seated; or they may never 'go off' the essential oil at all, in which case see 'Troubleshooting' on page 54. By the time your animal loses interest in oil you should see a significant reduction of the problem.

Interest levels will also vary depending on how serious the problem is. If the problem is minor, the response will be minimal with the animal sniffing the oil for a short time and being easily distracted from the oil. An animal who has an acute condition is likely to show very focussed interest over a few days, and one with a long-running problem may show sustained interest over a matter of weeks.

Interest levels are categorised as keen, moderate, or none. The level of interest dictates how often I offer the oil. When the interest is keen I offer the essential oils twice a day if I can. As interest diminishes I offer once a day. But don't worry, if you can't offer every day, the treatment will still work, even if the oils are only offered every few days

Keen interest

The main indicator of keen interest is that your animal will not be distracted from the oil, even if a noise catches her attention, she will quickly return to the essential oil.

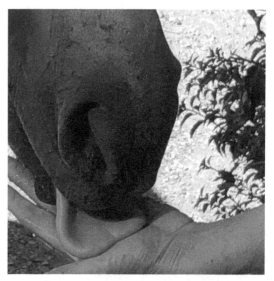

She may go into a deep trance with a lot of eye flickering, try to eat the bottle, or indicate an area of her body repeatedly and insistently, saying she wants the oil on her body.

If she takes the oil orally she will lick your hand firmly, possibly with the underside of the tongue (for more rapid penetration into the blood system).

Licking the oil with the underside of tongue, a sign of keen interest.

Moderate interest

In this response, an animal may take a sniff or lick of the oil, walk away to check out the surroundings, return for another sniff, walk away, return. He may also go into a light trance, or take a few licks from your hand, often around the oil rather than right on it. It is rare to see an animal ask for topical application when interest is moderate.

No interest

This is exactly what it says. The animal may take a sniff of the bottle, then immediately walk away. Horses will often clearly turn their heads away, or lower them below the bottle. Cats will leave the room in a hurry. My dear Gipsy would go to the other end of the garden as soon as she saw me going towards my oil bag if she had no interest in an oil.

Sometimes animals just need a day off from a certain oil, even setting up patterns where they want one oil one day and another the next. Only if they refuse the oil for three days in a row do I consider them finished with that oil and discontinue.

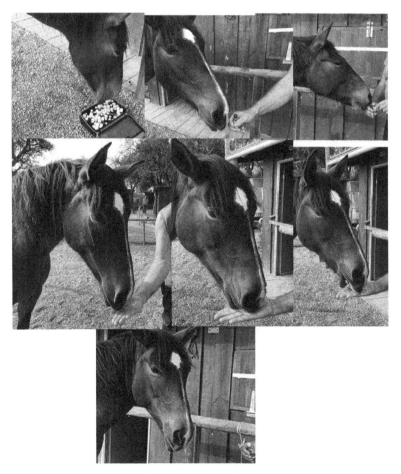

This is a sequence with a horse

HOW TO CHOOSE OILS FOR YOUR ANIMAL

Well, that's the general overview, now down to the nitty gritty: how do you choose the aromatics your animal needs? There are four easy steps to selecting the essential oil, hydrosol or vegetable oil your animal might need and then offering them to him to choose.

1. Setting your goal

This might seem obvious, but the more clearly you define what you perceive to be the problem, the easier it will be to choose oils. Think carefully about what you aim to achieve with the oils. The more you narrow your definition, the more obvious it will be which oils you need. If you say, "I want to make my dog feel good," you will have an endless list of possible oils. A clearer goal with more clues for matching the oil might be: "I want my dog to feel more confident, because since he was attacked as a youngster he always barks at strange dogs. I would also like to stop him getting an upset stomach when there are changes in his routine."

2. Choose an element

(You can skip this step if you choose to, but using Five Element Theory will refine your oil selection and your understanding of your animal.)

The next step is to decide which element your animal is, as this will help you define your oil choices further. So read through the section on the Five Elements in the next chapter, fill out the questionnaire, and decide which element most closely reflects your animal and his problems. Essential oils that match your animal's element are more likely to help him than those with similar properties that belong to another element.

3. Make your shortlist

Build a shortlist of five to seven essential oils by looking at Essential Oils for Specific Conditions (MA2) pages 98-108 in the Materia Aromatica. To get a more in-depth picture of the oils you are considering and see if they suit your animal, double check your oils using the Essential Oil Profiles (MA3). Use MA1, pages 92-97, to narrow your choices further till you have a few essential oils that match as many of your animal's character traits and symptoms as possible. Place oils that belong to the same element as your animal higher on your shortlist than those which match the problem but are of a different element.

Try to match the 'character' of the oil to the 'character' of the animal and its problem. E.g. If your animal has red, itchy skin, is nervous and highly strung, tends to get diarrhoea when upset, and is prone to having tantrums, find an essential oil that will take care of all those problems. In this case Roman chamomile would be a good match, especially if the animal is a Wood element. If your animal is Earth element, frankincense might be a better option.

4. Offer the oils for self-selection

Once you have a selection of essential oils, take the bottles to your animal, let him smell each one and see which ones he prefers. You can expect your animal to choose one central oil that he is particularly keen on, and two or three supporting oils that he may be less enthusiastic about, at least the first time they are offered.

For instance, if you want to choose oils for a horse with laminitis (a painful inflammation of the hoof lining, a common equine problem), look for essential oils to address the specific problems of this condition, in this case oils that will:

- » Reduce pain and inflammation, e.g. yarrow, plai, seaweed, rosemary, peppermint,
- » Support liver function, e.g. carrot seed, juniper berry, peppermint, seaweed, yarrow,
- » Increase circulation, e.g. rosemary, garlic, seaweed,
- » Lift the depression caused by pain/isolation, e.g. rose otto, neroli, or orange.

Oil selection made easy!

1. Set your therapeutic goal.
2. Decide your animal's element (optional)
3. In the Materia Aromatica, look through Essential Oils for Specific Conditions (MA2) and choose a few oils that are listed for the condition you are treating.
4. Cross reference the oils you have chosen in MA1 matching your therapeutic goal and your animal's history and character and decide on your shortlist, read individual profiles (MA4) if you want further clarification.
5. Allow your animal to smell each of the oils on your shortlist to choose what they need.

As you can see, some of the oils appear in several categories, which makes them more likely candidates for final selection. In this particular case I would expect the horse to choose seaweed, because it appears under so many categories, as well as an oil from each of the other categories. So the horse's final selection could be something like:

- » Seaweed, carrot seed, rosemary and orange, or
- » Seaweed, yarrow, juniper berry and neroli, or
- » Yarrow, plai, garlic and orange.

This is not to say that those are always going to be the choices of every horse, each situation is different and all factors must always be considered.

HOW TO OFFER AROMATICS FOR ANIMAL SELF-SELECTION

Having made your shortlist of essential oils, let your animal decide if the oils you have chosen are the ones he needs. Choose a quiet time, when there are no other distractions and remove other animals from the area, so the animal you want to treat can concentrate on you and the essential oils.

Horses and large animals

Allow your horse to smell the essential oils, one by one. Hold the open bottle firmly in your hand, so the neck of the bottle just peeps out, about a head's length away from the horse's nose.

It is important to give the horse space to come towards the oil if he chooses, do not push the bottle into his nose. Offer each bottle and see

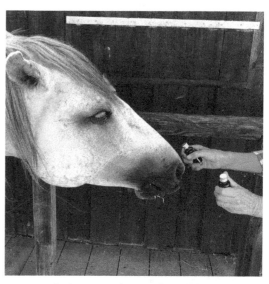

Let the horse stretch towards you, dont push the oils into her nose.

which ones he likes best. Once an animal has picked his oil(s)dilute each oil in a separate bottle, as per Table 1, page 52, then offer the diluted oils to the horse one by one, and follow his responses. Offer the oils once or twice a day until your horse loses interest.

Dogs

Once you have made your shortlist put the closed bottles of oils on the floor with a little space between them. Encourage your dog to smell them. Watch carefully and take note of those your dog sniffs more intently, or tries to lick.

Once he has found the oil he needs, he will stop sniffing. He might also try to pick up the bottle, so be prepared to stop him. Once he has chosen the oil(s), dilute each one in separate bottles as per Table 1, page 52, then offer each diluted oil and follow your animal's responses.

Offer the oils once or twice a day until your dog loses interest.

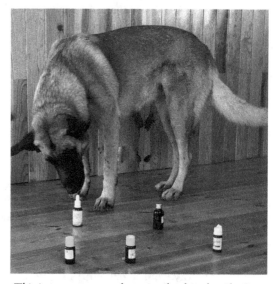

This is an easy way to let animals select the oils. Once you have made a shortlist put the bottles down and let the animal make her choice

Cats and small furries

It is best to use hydrosols with cats and small animals, (as explained later) but sometimes they need an essential oil as well. Make a shortlist. The smaller the animal the harder it is to spot their responses, as a small sniff, a quick lick of the tongue and staying near the bottle are considered positive responses.

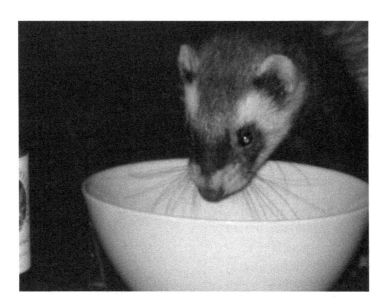

Calypso the ferret had a bald tail, we were not sure why. Here, she chooses witch hazel hydrosol, soothing, antiseptic and anti-haematoma. She nibbles the bottle top, so we put one drop in 50 ml of water and she takes a few licks, then curls up to sleep.

Once the oil/hydrosol is chosen, dilute essential oils as per Table 1, page 52, and hydrosols according to Table 4, page 64. Offer each selected solution one at a time and follow your animal's responses. Offer the oils once or twice a day until there is no further interest.

Wild, aggressive, or timid animals

Essential oils offer a perfect solution for working with undomesticated animals, feral cats or similar, and caged wild animals. Or those who do not wish to interact with humans any more, such as dogs who are fearful or aggressive because of bad experiences with humans. Because essential oils work through the olfactory system, you do not need to touch the animal or enter their personal space in order to treat them.

To work with a caged animal, stand outside the cage, far enough away not to provoke defensive behaviour from the animal. Open the bottle, stand or crouch in a non-threatening way and allow the animal to smell the oil. Keep an eye on his responses, but do not stare. If the animal is interested dilute the oil and smear some on a long pole or some other 'arm extension' and hold it out towards him. If this is too threatening then just put the oil on a plate and leave it in the cage for the animal to lick or sniff as it chooses. The last method does not work for primates however, as you do not want them to get the oil on their hands and then inadvertently rub their eyes. In this case stick with 'arm extensions' so you keep control of the oil.

Animals who are not caged, such as feral cats, can be encouraged to trust you, or at least be given the opportunity to help themselves, by leaving a saucer with diluted oils or hydrosols in a safe place for them to come to when they want.

Table 1: Animal responses and approximate dilutions of essential oils.

	Horses/large animals Do not offer more than 5 oils at one time.	Canines Do not offer more than three oils at one time.	Cats & small pets Hydrosols are safer than essential oils for cats.
Keen interest Offer twice a day	Smelling intently; lip curl (flehmen); follows the bottle; nibbles the bottle; trance.	Smells intently; licks lips or bottle; follows the aroma; rolls on back; lies down, head across paws; trance.	Smells intently; licks lips or bottle; follows the aroma; rolls on back; rubs against you; lies down in the room.
Moderate interest Offer once a day	Smells, looks away then smells again; ears forward; slightly flared nostrils; easily distracted.	A few sniffs then looks away or leaves, but then returns; keeps distance but stays in room; easily distracted.	One sniff then looks away but returns to the bottle; tongue licks quickly; easily distracted.
No interest Do not use	Turns away from the aroma; ears back; walks away.	Turns away from the aroma; one sniff and no further interest; tries to leave the room.	Leaves the room as you open the bottle.
Dilution Physical problem	3-5 drops essential oil in 5 ml of base oil.	2-3 drops of essential oil in 5 ml base oil.	1 drop essential oil in 10 ml base oil.
Dilution Emotional problem	1-3 drops essential oil in 5 ml of base oil.	1 drop essential oil in 5-10 ml of base oil.	1 drop essential oil to 10 –25 ml base oil.

BASIC RULES FOR SUCCESS

Patience

Patience is the most important aspect of offering essential oils. Choose a quiet time when you and your animal can focus on each other, unhurried and free of distractions. Do not offer oils if your animal is expecting to be fed or go out, and remove other animals from the area so they do not interfere.

Respect your animal's choice

It is very tempting for people, having made all that effort to choose the oils, to force the animal to participate. After all, we have a lifetime of conditioning that says WE know what is good for our animals. However, for safety and effectiveness, it is important you trust and respect the animal's wishes when using essential oils and truly listen to what is being communicated. If you force oils on your animal you risk creating an aversion at best, and an allergic reaction at worst.

Look at the whole picture

Another important key to success is looking at the problem holistically to see what else can be changed to reduce stress for the animal. This can include changes in diet, or changes in lifestyle; it could be as simple as changing the position of a bed (especially for cats), or as difficult as changing your own beliefs and habits.

Table 2: How to facilitate animal self-selection

Select a few oils and let your animal choose which ones he needs	Make a shortlist of possible oils. Allow your animal to smell each bottle of undiluted essential oil or hydrosol and choose which ones he likes. Keep the lid of the bottle on when offering to dogs, cats and small animals, lid off for equids and larger animals.
Assess the reaction	Assess your animal's reaction to the oils and dilute them as per Table 1.
Offer twice daily	Offer the essential oil to the animal twice a day, assessing his response each time and acting accordingly.
For as long as animal shows interest	Offer the oils for as long as the animal wants them and you are continuing to see an improvement, usually within two weeks.
Losing interest	When the animal shows no interest in an oil do not offer it for two to three days, then try again. If the animal still shows no interest, then he no longer needs that particular oil. THIS IS GOOD!
No loss of interest	If the animal still wants oils after two weeks re-assess. If the condition is improving, continue with oils. If no improvement: Check you have removed the cause of the problem; try different oils; spend quiet time together without the oils. Use hydrosols for on-going support in chronic conditions.

TROUBLESHOOTING

No interest

It sometimes happens that an animal will show no interest in the oils. There are several possible reasons for this, However, before you decide your animal does not want the oils, reassess your interpretation of the response. Make sure you are not mistaking a trance (a strong response) for 'no interest'.

In a trance, animals look as if they are sleeping with their eyes half open, often there is a flickering of the eyelids or twitching of the brow. Observe their nostrils carefully, if they are moving oil is being inhaled.

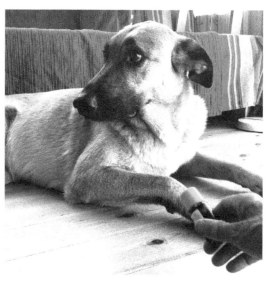

Bodhi looks worried as he turns his head away from the offered oil, this is a 'no'.

You can also change the order in which you offer the oils. Sometimes an animal needs to deal with an emotional issue before healing can start, so will need to have the oil for that issue before taking other oils, this is particularly true where there are issues of broken trust.

Another common reason for an animal to reject essential oils is if they are not diluted enough, particularly in the case of sensitive dogs, cats, and small animals. Dilute further by adding more base oil, then re-offer.

You may need to offer the oils a few times before the animal has enough confidence to interact with them, or he may just need tiny amounts at first as he regulates how much his body/mind can deal with. Or it could be that he feels no need for that essential oil. Or in the best scenario, he is totally healthy and doesn't need oils at all.

No loss of interest

Occasionally an animal does not lose interest in the oil. It is important to remember, an animal's desire for an essential oil is driven by the hedonic response, the desire for 'that which brings pleasure'. It is possible that the pleasure itself may become the goal; this can happen if an animal lives in a stressful environment. If you have not removed the original stressor from the animal's surrounding, he may still feel he needs oils.

If your animal's problem has resolved but he still wants the oils (this happens most commonly with dogs), it may be because he is enjoying the time spent with you listening. In this case, spend quiet time together without the oils.

The other reason an animal can show continued interest in an oil, is if he needs a second oil to completely resolve the problem. Offer some different oils. Once he has the exact oil he needs he should lose interest in the first one.

In Review

When using essential oils with animals, we allow them to select their own essential oils, hydrosols and base oils. The oil is diluted and offered to the animal twice a day to interact with. Within a few days or a week, or occasionally longer if it is a chronic physical problem, your four-legged friend will lose interest in the oil. You should see a clear improvement in the problem. If the problem has not cleared up check you removed stressors, then try offering other essential oils. Simple!

Table 3: The main reasons for no interest in the oils

Reason	Solution
You have the wrong oils for the problem.	Choose new oils.
The root cause of the problem has not been removed, for instance a poor diet or stressors in her environment, or a painful back (although this more usually makes them want to take the oils forever).	Remove stressors.
The animal does not feel safe enough in her environment to take the oils and start healing.	Offer angelica root or rose, 1 drop to 5 ml of base oil. Work on building animal's trust.
If the animal is constitutionally not suited to essential oils and would prefer hydrosols or homeopathy.	Try hydrosols.
The oil needs to be diluted more.	Dilute by 50%.
There is nothing wrong with the animal as far as she is concerned. This can be because she really is healthy or the problem is being controlled by conventional medicine, such as steroids.	Rejoice! Your animal feels fine! If your animal is on long-term medication such as pain killers or steroids, consult with your vet before making any changes.

SAFETY

Essential oils are relatively safe to use, especially if you allow the animals to guide you, but as with any active substance you must understand the material and follow some basic rules.

Essential oils are not natural!

Within every plant there is a system of checks and balances to buffer harsher chemicals. When using essential oils we must remember they are man-made! When we separate the essential oil from the plant, we remove it from any natural buffers, not least the bulk of plant matter. In the wild, an animal's stomach would be full, long before he overdosed on essential oil. We must use essential oils as nature intended, well diluted.

Always dilute

Essential oils should be used in high dilutions and topical use should be kept to a minimum. Never offer undiluted oils to a dog or cat as the power of the aroma can seem like an assault to them. Keep the bottle closed when offering first selection.

Request permission

Allow your animals to smell EACH oil before EACH application. To apply oils without offering them first is at best annoying (imagine being smothered in a perfume you hated with no way to wash it off) and at worst dangerous. The only recorded cases of animals having adverse reactions to essential oils are when the oils have been added to their food, strapped onto their nose in an inhaler, or put on their skin.

A few basic rules for safety

> » Dilute essential oils well in a good quality base oil or water-based gel before use.
> » In the unlikely event of your animal showing a reaction such as skin irritation or shortness of breath, discontinue use immediately and contact a vet or professional therapist.
> » Store essential oils in a cool, dark place with their caps firmly closed.
> » Never leave essential oil bottles in reach of animals: horses have been known to eat them, dogs have stolen them from counter tops!
> » Do not use on pregnant animals or allow pregnant women to offer the oils.
> » Pay attention to the cautions and safety issues with each essential oil.
> » If your animal is still interested in oils after two weeks, contact a professional for advice.

An extra word on safety for cats

Cats lack an important detoxification process present in most other mammals, so are easily poisoned. A cat's liver has limited ability to metabolize terpenes. Most essential oils contain a complex assortment of mono and sesqui-terpenes, but in particular, avoid oils containing phenols when working with cats.

Many cat owners report that when they smell of essential oil their cat will attack them, or lick them frantically. This can lead people to believe their cat really loves essential oil, when, in fact, it is literally driving them crazy as it overloads their neural network. Cats can also behave as they do with catnip (after all it is the essential oil in catnip they are responding to) jumping around and having a mad moment or five.

There have been reports of cats dying after exposure to essential oils, but to my knowledge, all recorded cases of death were due to misuse or overuse of essential oils. For example, topical application of undiluted tea tree oil, which despite its widespread use is not safe for cats. The feline liver needs 48 hours to process and excrete terpenes, so frequent exposure to low quantities of essential oil can also cause toxicity. Make sure your cat can leave the room when you diffuse essential oils or burn aroma candles.

There is no need to be hysterical about keeping essential oils away from cats - after all, the natural world is full of essential oil and the genus Felis survives perfectly well. However, I recommend the use of hydrosols rather than essential oils for cats.

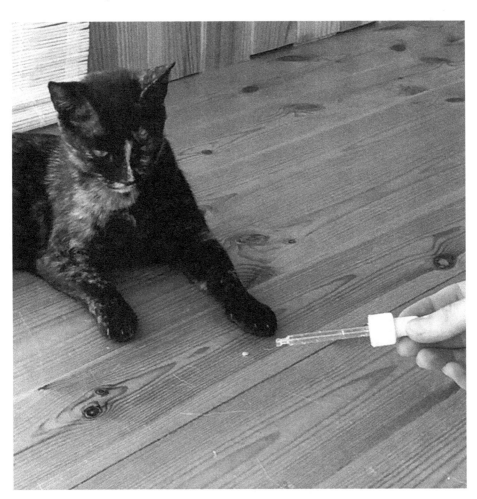

CARRIER OILS: A GOOD BASE

The right oil for the job

Essential oils always need to be diluted in a carrier oil, also known as a base oil. This can be pure, cold-pressed vegetable oil or vegetable oil that has been infused with healing herbs, known as macerated, infused or herbal oil.

Choosing a base oil specifically for the presenting condition is important, as the right base oil enhances the essential oils and creates an even more holistic remedy.

For instance, if you have chosen essential oils for an animal with arthritis, you can dilute them in hemp seed or St John's wort oil, both of which are good for arthritis. When the animal's problem is emotional the best choice is often a 'neutral' vegetable oil that has little healing activity of its own, such as grapeseed.

Animals must be allowed to choose the vegetable and herbal oils they need just as they choose the essential oil. Base oils can also be used without the essential oils, in which case they work like a food supplement, but still allow them to choose.

What's in an oil?

Vegetable oils are extracted from the nuts or seeds of a variety of plants. For therapeutic purposes, use high quality, cold-pressed vegetable oils, preferably organic, as pesticides and other chemicals can easily be carried through in the extraction process to contaminate the oil. Don't use highly processed supermarket oils, except in emergency.

> ### What is cold pressed oil?
>
> You may well have heard that cold pressed is superior, but why? And what does it mean? Cold-pressed oil is obtained through pressing and grinding fruit or seeds. Traditonally this was done with heavy granite millstones. Nowadays. Commercial operation use stainless steel presses. Pressing and grinding produces heat through friction, but in Europe the temperature must not rise above 120°F (49°C) for oil to be considered cold pressed. In the USA it is unregulated. Cold pressed oils retain all of their flavour, aroma, and nutritional value and do not contain trans-fatty acids.

Herbal oil, also known as macerated or infused oil, is made by soaking the flowers and/or leaves of the herb in (usually) sunflower or olive oil. After two to six weeks the oil is drained off and filtered. This process draws the heavy, fat-soluble molecules of the plant into the oil. These heavier molecules are lost in the process of distilling essential oils, so combining essential oil with these macerated herbal oils is a little like putting the whole plant back together.

Quality and safety

Good quality carrier oils have not been heated anywhere in their production process; organic, cold-pressed oils should be your standard. Macerated oils should be made with pesticide free herbs. Carrier oils vary in stability: hemp seed, flax seed and rosehip start to deteriorate after about three months, while jojoba, one of the most stable carriers, lasts at least two years.

Choosing a base oil

Choose a base oil for your animal the same way you choose an essential oil, look at all the available information and match your animal's symptoms and character to the oil. Select a base oil that complements and supports your healing intention. Then check that your animal likes the oil. You can offer up to three carrier oils to your animal and see which one he selects, in the same way you offer essential oils.

Hold a bottle in each hand and let the animal smell each one, then widen the distance between the bottles and see which one your animal moves toward more keenly. If you have more than two oils, offer the oil he chose the first time and the oil that you have not yet offered, and compare the animal's response between the two oils. Repeat this process until you are sure which one he has picked. Once your animal has chosen a base oil, add each of the chosen essential oils to its own bottle of the base oil.

Why dilute essential oils?

I am often asked if it is really necessary to dilute essential oils. The answer is yes, unless you are a fully trained animal aromatherapist because:

Using distilled essential oils is not what nature intended. In their natural state essential oils are highly diluted by the bulk of the plant matter in which they are found, they make up a very small percentage of the active ingredients.

Diluted essential oils are safe, effective and economical for every animal guardian to use, the only person who gains by using more essential oil than is necessary is your supplier.

You wouldn't use four pain killers when two will do the job, same with essential oils, too much of a good thing can be harmful.

HYDROSOLS: THE HEALING POWER OF WATER

The gentle healer

I have mentioned hydrosols in passing, now it is time to get to know them a little better. I have found hydrosols work synergistically with essential oils and give an extra dimension to my work.

The gentle energetic quality of hydrosols often works on a more etheric level than essential oils, clearing trauma that is caught in the auric field (the energy field that surrounds the physical body). Sensitive animals, who find essential oils too direct, often respond very well to hydrosols.

First, a little background

The distilling of aromatic plants is an ancient tradition, especially in the Middle East where every home had a still to make food flavourings and medicines. It is quite possible that essential oils used to be considered a by-product of the hydrosol, rather than the other way round.

Nonetheless, until recently hydrosols were seen by aromatherapists as a waste product of the distillation process with minimal therapeutic value. Luckily for us hydrosols are now enjoying a renaissance.

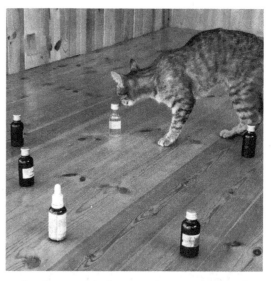

It is best to use hydrosols with cats, young, small, or frail animals.

So, what is a hydrosol?

Hydrosol, also known as hydrolat or flower water, is a by- or co-product of the distillation process of essential oils. When essential oils are distilled the steam is gathered in a condenser. The essential oil is collected in a Florentine flask and the steam (now water) flows into a vat. This water, the hydrosol, contains heavier, water-soluble molecules that did not evaporate, as well as tiny traces of essential oil, so hydrosols are healing in their own right, but much gentler than essential oil.

Both the action and fragrance of hydrosols is gentler than essential oils. The scent lacks the penetrative power of essential oil and has a much heavier herbal note, which can be almost unpleasant. Sometimes the smell is quite different from the essential oil, for example, frankincense or yarrow.

There are some plants which do not produce enough essential oil to gather but are distilled for the hydrosol, such as **witch hazel** (*Hamamelis virginiana*) or **cornflower (Centaurea cyanus)**.

Aromatic Waters

Aromatic waters are similar to hydrosols but are distilled for the water itself, the essential oils are not removed. Because they are considered a primary product they are usually distilled at lower heat, bringing over more active constituents. They can be used in the same way as hydrosols, but may need more dilution.

The chemistry of hydrosols

Hydrosols are relatively new to the world of modern aromatherapy and the chemical structure has not been analysed to the same degree as essential oils, so most hydrosols do not have chemical monographs.

We do know that hydrosols contain water-soluble elements of a plant and some volatile oils. However, the chemical make-up of essential oil found in hydrosol differs from that which is separated, containing more of the gentle alcohols and a very low ratio of ketones and other harsh components.

Cheers!

Just as with essential oils, if you are going to use hydrosols then get to know them personally. Suzanne Catty suggests pouring a little hydrosol into a wine glass, which is designed to enhance the aromatics of wine. This way you can examine how the hydrosol looks, what colour and viscosity it is, whether it has a 'slick' of oil on the surface and other visible features. You can then swirl it like a wine taster to encourage the aroma to rise and examine the smell and taste. This way you know what is normal for a hydrosol and will notice if it starts to 'turn'. The colour and taste also give you clues as to how the hydrosol can help you as per the Chinese Five Element theory (see Chapter 3).

Quality control

As with essential oils – and perhaps even more so – the quality of hydrosols is highly variable. Because hydrosols are still often seen as a by-product of essential oils, distillers do not always pay attention to the quality of the hydrosol, seeing it as a waste product from which they can make a little extra cash. This is changing, and will change even more as the interest in hydrosols as a healing product increases. Which is why, when possible I prefer to buy hydrosols (aromatic waters) that have been distilled as the primary product.

Just like essential oils, the quality of hydrosols can vary according to distillation methods and which part of the water is collected. It is generally accepted that the best hydrosol is the first 30% of the distillation. Collecting more than that dilutes the active constituents with heavier non-water soluble molecules. The purity of the water used in the distillation process will also affect the quality of the hydrosol.

Safety and storage

The average shelf life of an unpreserved hydrosol is eight months to two years, depending on pH level (the lower the pH the longer they last). Hydrosols should be stored in a cool place, preferably in glass bottles. It is better not to keep them refrigerated if possible, as condensation from the change in temperature when you put htem in and out of the fridge can cause bacterial growth.

Take care not to contaminate them by breathing into the bottle, putting your fingers on the inside of the lid or the opening of the bottle. Hydrosols sold in shops must have a standard preservative added by law in the European Union, this is usually a small amount of ethyl alcohol.

According to Suzanne Catty, who has written a seminal book on the use of hydrosols, "Hydrosols: the Next Aromatherapy", you can monitor the purity and quality of hydrosols by testing the pH level, which varies from hydrosol to hydrosol but is generally 5.5 or below. The hydrosol becomes less acidic (the pH level increases) as it starts to deteriorate. By monitoring the pH of your hydrosols you can have early warning of when they start to go 'off'. Test the pH of your hydrosols when you receive them, and then monthly to see if the pH changes.

As hydrosols start to deteriorate they become cloudy and the smell turns musty, at this stage you can use them for domestic cleaning purposes (well I do, nothing like a litre of lavender water down the loo!), or pass them through a coffee filter to clean them up, and use them in your bath.

Internal use of hydrosols, is generally considered to be safe. However, there are some who are concerned about internal use due to the relative sparseness of information and concerns about bacterial contamination.

Actually, the acidity of the hydrosol inhibits bacterial growth and I have not had problems using them internally on myself or with animals. However, it is crucial to use a good quality product and monitor your hydrosols for bacterial growth.

When to use hydrosols

A moving story

Moving house can be a stressful time for any animal. If the move involves flying it is even more intimidating for animal and owner. I have used hydrosols many times to help reduce the stress of travel. One week before the move add one drop of 3x solution of frankincense or neroli to everything you or your animals drink, this stops stress building up. For the journey itself, you will need a bottle of 1x solution of valerian hydrosol and your 3x frankincense or neroli. Give them as much as they want of the hydrosols straight from the pipette. If your animal has to travel in the hold of a plane, supply two water bottles (the ones used for hamster/rabbit cages work well, but make sure your pet knows how to use it). Fill one bottle with plain water and one with valerian, frankincense or neroli hydrosol diluted appropriately.

Hydrosols are a gentler plant extract so they can be used instead of essential oils where the oils might be too harsh. Use them in place of the essential oil of the same plant, for animals that are young, or weak, for cats and small animals, for wild animals, or for long term care.

Unlike essential oils, hydrosols are water-soluble so can be added to water and left out for animals to self-medicate as they wish. This is particularly useful for herds of animals, wild animals, or animals who do not want to interact with humans.

For instance, you can add ¼ cup of rose hydrosol to large tub of water and leave it in the lambing shed, so all the ewes have access to it after giving birth if they choose. You must also provide a source of clean, fresh water as well.

You can also use hydrosols alongside essential oils, particularly for the emotional aspect of a problem, and especially for deep-rooted emotional problems that may even be genetic, or 'constitutional', part of the animal's basic make-up.

In many cases you can use hydrosol to replace some of the useful but expensive essential oils such as rose otto *(Rosa damascena)* or melissa *(Melissa officinalis)*.

I find hydrosols a safe and easy solution when an animal needs on-going support for a chronic condition, as they are much less likely to provoke sensitisation than essential oils.

Another advantage of hydrosols is that many of them can be used near and in the eyes as washes. Hydrosols can also be used in place of water when making up topical treatments such as gels and clays.

Table 4: Dilutions and dosage for hydrosols

	Initial dilution	Horse/large animals	Dogs	Cats/small animals	Birds
Acute physical problem	Undiluted	10-30ml in bucket of water	10-50 drops in 100 ml water	3-10 drops in 100 ml water	3-4 drop in 50 ml water
Chronic physical problem	Undiluted or 1x	10 drops in bucket of water	1-20 drops in 100 ml water	1 pipetter 1x or 1-10 drops in 50 ml water	1 pipette 1 x
Emotional problem	1x	10 drops in bucket of water	1-10 drop in 100 ml water	1-10 drops in 50 ml water	1 drop in teaspoon water
Shock/trauma	undiluted	Up to 10 drops on tongue	1-3 drops on tongue	offer to smell 1 drop on paw or ears	1-2 drops on beak

Selecting hydrosols

The basic principle of allowing your animal to select his remedy still applies to hydrosol (or herbs). To choose a hydrosol, make your shortlist based on character and symptoms just as with essential oil.

Once the animal has made her selection, dilute the hydrosols according to the chart below. I generally start with a few drops in a saucer of water and either add more drops of hydrosol or more water, depending on the animal's reaction. Cats will pull a face if the dilution is too strong, or sniff and search if the dilution is not strong enough.

Add the hydrosols to water and place in a convenient location, preferably not near your pet's food, as you want to monitor how often they go to the bowl. Put down fresh hydrosol each day for as long as the animal shows interest. Always provide fresh clean drinking water as well.

Homeopathic hydrosol

Hydrosols can be diluted down to 'homeopathic' solutions. I have found these effective for deep-seated problems, such as phobias, constitutional nervousness, or if emotions are a strong factor in the problem. For instance, homeopathic valerian works well for fear of fireworks. I use these solutions where many people use Bach flower remedies. Most commonly I use what I call a 1x solution, one drop of hydrosol in 30 ml of distilled or spring water. I then bang the bottom of the bottle on the palm of my hand one hundred times. This activates and energises the remedy. You can then take one drop of this solution and repeat the process to make a 2x solution, and again to make 3x. Add drops to water or use undiluted.

Case study: Flora the fearful fox-hound

Flora was a foxhound bitch, who found herself in the care of the RSPCA. No-one knew why, but she was terrified of people, leaving her pen or socialising. When people came to her kennel she would cower in the corner so her chances of adoption were slim. I was asked to help her with essential oils. The oils chosen were frankincense to counteract fearfulness, angelica root for reconnecting with herself and feeling protected, rose for self acceptance and to heal resentful anger arising from past abuse.

As I approached the bars of her kennel she ran to the back and hid. I crouched down outside the bars, opened the frankincense and waited patiently; I could feel she was drawn to the oil. Without looking at her, I stretched my arm towards her with the bottle in my hand. Very slowly she inched towards me until she was about 2 metres away, then she lay down and breathed deeply.

After some minutes she stood up, stretched and moved to the back of her kennel. I repeated the process with the other two oils. With each oil she approached more confidently, The angelica she sniffed quickly. The rose she smelled deeply then disappeared inside her hideaway.

I left hydrosols with the staff to dilute in water and leave in her kennel, so she could self-medicate. A week later I received a note from the centre manager, who had been away on holiday when Flora started her treatment. She told me how surprised and delighted she had been to find Flora in reception greeting visitors on her return to work.

"Our task must be to free ourselves... by widening our circle of compassion to embrace all living creatures and the whole of nature and its beauty."

- Albert Einstein

CHAPTER 3

FIVE ELEMENTS FOR ANIMAL WELL-BEING

Why Five Element Theory?

I have found the Five Element Theory really helpful when it comes to choosing which essential oil or hydrosol an animal needs, because it gives me an insight into an animal's character, behaviour and possible health problems. I use the principles all the time to care for my own animals.

I also use the Five Elements to help me understand which food will best suit an animal, how he prefers to learn, and other useful keys for happy living. You don't have to use this theory for choosing essential oils, but it does help pick the best oil for the job and get to the root of a problem.

What is Five Element Theory?

The Five Element Theory is a part of Traditional Chinese Medicine (TCM). It is a way of understanding the causes and manifestations of physical and emotional problems in humans and animals, and emphasises the need to heal the emotions in order to heal the body.

Five Element Theory is based on the cycles of nature. The five elements are Water, Wood, Fire, Earth and Metal, elements of nature that are seen to nourish and control each other.

Everything, including humans and animals, is made up of all the elements, and moves through all the elements in a lifetime. However, an individual is said to have a 'constitutional type' aligned strongly with one or other of the elements and is likely to show character traits, physical problems, and emotional responses specific to that type.

Five phases

The Five Element Theory is also known as The Five Phases, because it is based on the observation of nature's rhythms and phases. These phases can be considered a map of the flow of energy that governs us all, the phases we all pass through in our life. Everything in the universe can be ascribed to the rule of one element or another, and each element is said to 'rule' a whole set of functions (see Tables 5 & 6, pages 74/75). Each of us has an essential affinity to one element or another, known as a constitutional type, and we are likely to express patterns of illness and behaviour that are related to that element. For example, an Earth type is likely to worry about things a lot and have problems with digestion. A Metal type might suffer from asthma and be somewhat aloof.

However, that is not to say that we are exclusively one element. You cannot say, 'I am Earth' in the same way you can say, 'I am a Taurus'. We are made up of all the elements and move through them all in the phases of our life. For example, when we are young and full of 'get up and go' we are expressing Wood energy, as we grow old and our hair turns grey and bones become weaker, this is Water having its way with us. Each day can also be divided into five phases as well: morning, noon, afternoon, evening and night.

Choosing oils for a Wood horse

Max is a 24-year-old Quarter horse gelding who is intermittently lame due to past tendon injuries. He was once a champion but is now semi-retired, used only for some light riding. He has not taken well to retirement and can seem depressed at times, especially if he is in his stable for too long. When out riding he acts as if angry and frustrated, lashing out at other horses if they come too close. His owners want to help him feel happier in his new lifestyle and to prevent any recurrence of the lameness.

His history & behaviour suggests Max is a Wood type: he was a champion; damaged tendons; doesn't like retirement; he gets depressed when shut in his stable; angry/frustrated when ridden. So my shortlist favours Wood oils. Max chose: bergamot, carrot seed (animals can view retirement as abandonment) and yarrow. I now consider a base oil. On my shortlist are: comfrey oil, whose green colour makes it Woody, and carrot oil, which is reparative and nourishing to the liver. Max chose the carrot oil. I then diluted 3-5 drops of each essential oil in its own 5 ml bottle of carrot oil. Max initially intereacted with each of the oils,losing interest over about 10 days as he felt better.

The elements are inter-dependent, if one element has too much or too little energy it will eventually effect all the other elements. When energy is flowing smoothly through all the cycles we call it 'health'. In this state, no individual element is more obvious than the next and each one is expressed naturally. When there is a blockage or an imbalance in the flow of energy, we can see an element more clearly as it manifests in physical or emotional problems.

CREATION AND CONTROL

In nature, one thing feeds another, and so it is in the Five Element Theory, each element feeds, or is the 'parent' of the one that follows it in the circle. In the Creation cycle Water nourishes Wood and Wood feeds Fire's flames, the ash of Fire becomes Earth and Earth creates Metal in its bowels, the minerals from Metal leach into Water to enrich it, and on it goes. But rampant growth would lead to destruction; an excess of Fire razes the forest and exhausts its Wood supply while drying up all the Water!

So we have a Control cycle where Water controls Fire, Wood controls Earth, Fire controls Metal, Earth controls Water, and Metal controls Wood, like the spokes of a bicycle keeping the wheel round. Look at the Cycle of Creation (the outer arrows) and the Cycle of Control (the inner arrows) in the diagram below and start to get a sense of the dynamic flow that is the nature of the Five Phases.

The Five Elements: relationships and characteristics

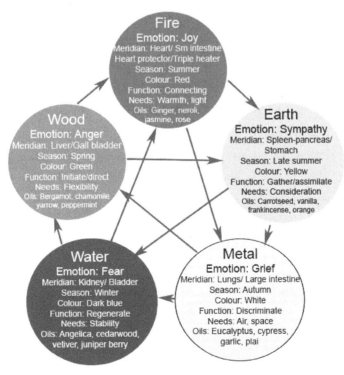

Imbalances in the flow of energy can show up through the Creation cycle if the 'parent' element lacks energy to feed its 'child', or if the energy is stuck in one element and not flowing on. Or the imbalance could be due to too much or too little Control. Wherever the problem starts it is likely to come out in the element that is generally weakest. If at this stage the problem is not taken care of it will eventually impact the health of each element and we will see health or behaviour problems arising.

THE ELEMENTS RULE!

Each element 'rules' a range of things within the body, including: a pair of meridians, an emotion, a climate condition, certain body tissues, a body part, physical, emotional and spiritual functions. Knowing which element rules which function is one of the keys to grasping the Five Element Theory and being able to use it to choose oils for your animal. Tables 5 and 6 (page 74/75) list some of the characteristics that are ruled by each element and how the element will manifest when balanced and when out of balance. Take some time to study the charts and see if you can recognise which element you are seeing in animals and people that you know.

The more balanced a person/animal is, the less you will see one particular element. Also, it is possible that as your animal comes into balance you will see different aspects of his character as the dominant element allows the other ones to express themselves.

Recognising elemental patterns

Based on the information in Tables 5 and 6 you can start to read the patterns that would indicate that you are seeing the influence of one particular element clearly. If you see one element particularly strongly choose oils to balance that element. This is a simplistic way of using the Five Elements, but is effective with essential oils because of their wide range of actions. So, if your animal has a skin problem and you see a lot of Earth indicators, you would choose frankincense or carrot seed, oils that have a strong connection to Earth, not yarrow, a more Wood centred oil.

Feel, don't think

Using the Five Elements is an intuitive art that is somewhat subjective. Try to catch the feeling of what is being expressed and do not think about it too hard. The more you observe the world through the prism of the Five Elements, putting theory into practice, the easier it becomes.

IDENTIFYING YOUR ANIMAL'S ELEMENT

Having read the charts you are sure to have some thoughts on which element your animal most closely reflects. You might feel confused because your animal fits many of the categories, but it is normal and desirable that we reflect aspects from all of the elements, as they are all present within us all. The more balanced we are the less any one element will stick out.

Disappearing elements

When I first met Star I was struck by her good looks, but she was very shut down, and in her own world. Despite this she gave a feeling of warmth and softness to anyone who touched her. I put her down as Fire, based on her looks, warmth & her ability to 'check out' & take herself away mentally, a Heart Protector defence mechanism. Two years of sensitive handling by a loving owner, life in a herd of horses, and quantities of essential oil later, it is very hard to see any single element when I look at Star. She looks & acts more like an Earth horse, kind, reliable, with a round belly, loves nothing more than eating, but she is also able to express a Fiery playful side, has the politeness of Metal, the initiative of Wood and the cautiousness of Water, when each is appropriate.

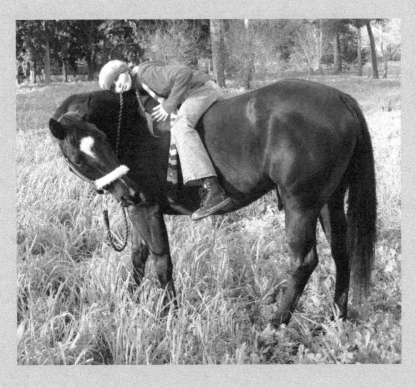

With humans there are various indicators which help a practitioner choose an element:

» Observation, particularly colour of the complexion and tongue

» Listening to the sound of the voice, paying attention to tone and HOW questions are answered.

» Smell of the breath and body

» Touch (assessing temperature and texture) and checking the pulses.

With animals, I focus on:

» The physical appearance,

» How they feel to the touch,

» How they smell,

» How they react to stimuli and situations.

» Sometimes an animal's voice will reveal them as well. A small dog with a particularly aggressive 'shout' of a bark could indicate Wood, as would a dog or horse that has no shout at all

» What the guardian says.

A complete lack of the emotion representing the element is a strong indicator, meaning, an animal who lacks fear to the point of recklessness could well be Water element.

Expanding the circle

The Five Elements are like a never-ending Russian doll, the pattern repeating over and over; each circle in the circle containing five circles, ad infinitum.

In the case of animals, each breed or species could be categorised as belonging to an Element. For instance, we could say dogs are Wood, as their primary motivation in life is the hunt (go-getters), and they must be innovative and disciplined to succeed; horses are Fire, they signify freedom, connectedness and warmth; cats are Water, wise, solitary, self-sufficient.

Then we can break it down further into breeds: Labradors, with their love of food and family are Earth, Jack Russell terriers are Wood, individualists that go rushing into any challenge with gusto; Arabian horses are Fire, highly-strung, reactive, curious; cob-types are Earth, steady and reliable. When assessing an individual, look past these generalities and ask, is he calm *for an Arabian*, or greedy *for a Labrador*.

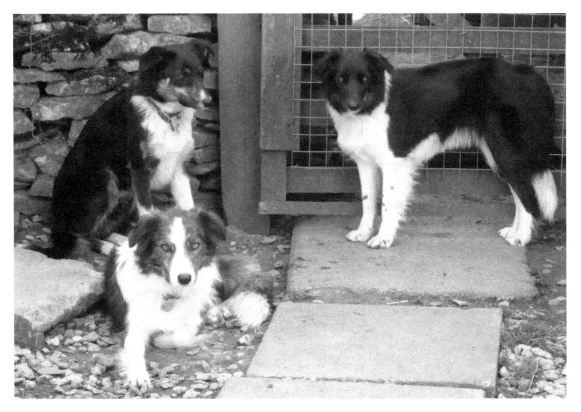

Elemental Examples: These border collies are siblings, yet each one displays a different element type. Molly, on the right, is Wood, sharp intense eyes, always ready to work, with a tendency to be too aggressive with the sheep. Zed, sitting, is Metal, he is a very good boy, easily offended by impolite behaviour, and a conscientious worker. Doug, Mr Fire, connecting with us even here, is charming, loves human contact and hates being left alone.

USING FIVE ELEMENT THEORY TO CHOOSE ESSENTIAL OILS

As interesting as the Five Element Theory is, and as varied its applications, the main purpose for its appearance in this book is to help you choose the best essential oil for your animal.

Each essential oil can be related to a specific element by their fragrance and their actions, or more usually two or three elements. Animals with Wood characteristics are more likely to respond to a Wood oil; if they are showing characteristics of Wood and Earth you can choose an essential oil that is both Wood and Earth.

So, once you have figured out which element you are seeing most strongly in your animal choose an oil that reflects that element, and treats the physical and emotional symptoms you are seeing. Not all the oils you choose have to belong to your chosen element, but they might be primarily Earth, say, with Metal and Water as secondary elements (the ones that are written in brackets).

FIVE ELEMENT PERSONALITY TYPES

Five Element Theory helps us read our animals better and understand why they respond to situations in a certain way, which food is good for them, which training method they would prefer and which essential oils they need. It can also clarify the dynamic of the relationship between you and your animal.

Both you and your animal are mainly influenced by a particular element, so in understanding how the elements relate to each other in the Control and Creation cycles you can recognise the dynamic of the relationship between you. For example, if you are a 'get up and go' Wood type who likes action and adventure but tends to burn out and get depressed, you are likely to be frustrated by a relationship with a stay-at-home Earth type who loves routine and likes to keep everyone happy; and the Earth type will be stressed by trying to keep you happy and calm.

Below are descriptions of the five personality types and how you can best support their physical, emotional and spiritual needs.

Table 5: The Five Elements Rule

	Metridians/ organ	Emo- tion	Season	Climate	Time	Sound	Body parts	Colour
Wood 'Growth'	Liver/Gall bladder	Anger	Spring	Wind	11p.m to 3 a.m.	Shout	Eyes, nails, tendons, ligaments,	Green
Fire 'Connection'	Heart/ Small intestine, Heart protector/triple warmer	Joy	Sum- mer	Heat	11a.m to 3 p.m	Laugh	Blood, vessels, tongue, complex- ion	Red
Earth 'Gath- ering	Spleen-pancre- as/Stomach	Sympa- thy	Late Sum- mer	Damp	7-11 a.m	Sing	Muscles, mouths, lips	Ochre
Metal 'Separation'	Lungs/large Intestine	Grief	Au- tumn	Dryness	3-7 a.m	Cry	Skin, nose, body hair	White
Water 'Survival'	Kidney/Bladder	Fear	Winter	Cold	3-7 p.m	Groan	Ears, bone, head hair	Dark blue

Table 6: Keys to understanding the Five Elements

	Wood	Fire	Earth	Metal	Water
In Balance	Easy-going, motivated, organised.	Self-aware, sensitive, joyful, well-integrated.	Thoughtful, caring, supportive.	Communicative vital, positive.	Determined, resourceful, astute.
Excess	Tense, frustrated, rigid, compulsive.	Exciteable, agitated, hyper-sensitive, scattered.	Anxious, worried, neurotic concern for others.	Brittle, aloof, defensive, melancholic.	Restless, reckless, driven.
Deficient	Depressed, lethargic, grumpy.	Despondent, timid, collapsed.	Confused, no concentration, emotionally demanding.	Loss of instincts, no initiative.	Apathetic, overwhelmed, fearful.
Typical character	Likes action, adventure, thrives on challenge, easily bored, hates confinement, can be impatient, or bad tempered.	Confident, loves intimacy, playful, likes to be centre of attention even if shy, oversensitive to other's moods.	Agreeable, wants to be needed, seeks togetherness, predictable, likes routine, can be lazy, slow to learn, stubborn.	Likes structured environment, respects authority, sets high standards for self & others, polite, exaggerated or lacking sense of personal space.	Self-contained, introspective, reserved, philosophical, suspicious, slow to make friends, loyal.
Likely problems	Intolerance, mood swings, high blood pressure, inflamed nerves, tendon problems, sciatica, neck tension, irritated eyes, irritable bowel, compulsive behaviour.	Excema, arrhythmia, low blood pressure, intolerant of cold or heat, circulatory problems, extreme shyness, over-exciteability.	Obesity, swollen glands, water retention, lymphodoema, digestive problems, poor muscle tone, obsessive thinking, fungal infections, food obsession.	Asthma, constipation, stiff joints, dry skin/hair, environmental sensitivities, defensive aggression, poor communication skills.	Sclerosis, arthritis, teeth /bone problems, hypersensitive hearing or deafness, no sex drive, weak back, urinary problems, phobias, fear aggression.
Healing Energy	Patience, encouragement.	Affection, playfulness.	Nurture, routine.	Space, order.	Reassurance, quietness.
Essential oils	Bergamot, chamomile. helichrysum.	Neroli, rose, ginger.	Fennel, benzoin Lemon.	Eucalyptus, cypress, garlic.	Cedarwood, angelica root, juniper berry.

WATER - THE PHILOSOPHER

» Meridians: Kidney/Bladder

» Season: Winter

» Climate: Cold

» Time of day: Night

» Emotion: Fear

» Fed by Metal, controlled by Earth, controls Fire

Physical appearance: Strong, dense, lean physique, although can be fleshy; sculptured face, high forehead, long narrow head, deep set eyes; broader at hips; long sensitive toes/feet that often appear large for their body size; thick glossy coats and manes/tails; flowing movement.

Key clues: Large boned, large feet for size, remarkably glossy coat, very deep melting eyes.

Feel to Touch: Yielding but firm.

Motivating force: Survival.

They value: Clarity.

They hate: Noise and commotion.

Most likely to find them: Alone in a quiet corner thinking deep thoughts.

Water types are canny and solitary by nature tending to keep their thoughts and feelings to themselves and are inherently sensitive souls. They like to take care of themselves and do not put their trust in others lightly. They are large-boned but graceful, with lustrous coats and clear eyes that can appear to see right into you. They are very loyal but have a tendency to keep apart from the world, relying on others to draw them out of themselves.

Out of balance they can become isolated in themselves and harden, appearing crusty and cynical. Once they retreat too far they become fearful and despondent, grouchy and over-sensitive, losing all sense of themselves. They find it hard to trust in the judgement of others, and may display fear or anxiety under pressure as they need time to evaluate situations. They are likely to suffer from cold, bone problems, bad back, kidney or bladder problems, sensitive hearing, fearfulness, and an extreme 'flight' impulse.

In essence: Self-sufficient and resilient, Water types are survivors, but because they are basically highly sensitive they may cut themselves off to survive, acting fearfully when we try to connect with them. Once they trust you they are true partners.

They need: Warmth, but not to be fussed over; a respect for their space and understanding of their sensitivity; to learn in their own good time. They are likely to need mineral supplementation.

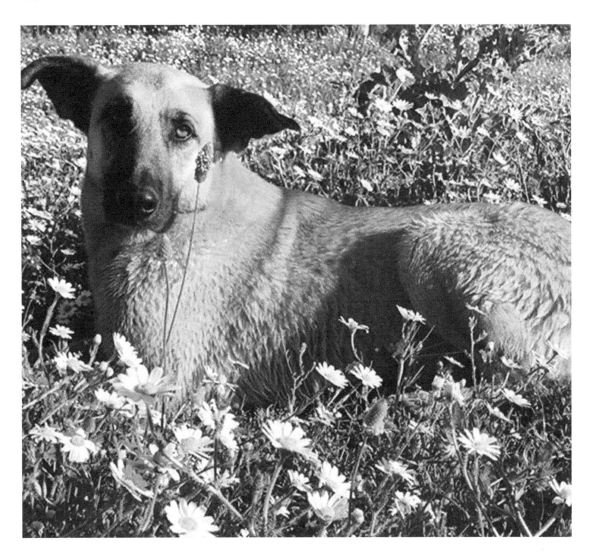

WOOD - THE ADVENTURER

- » Meridians: Liver/Gall bladder
- » Season: Spring
- » Climate: Wind
- » Time of day: Early morning
- » Emotion: Anger
- » Feeds Fire, controlled by Metal, controls Earth

Physical appearance: Muscular, square physique, yet quite lean. They move quickly and easily and yet can sometimes look stiff or wooden. They tend to have thick, coarse skin/coats, strong, slim, sinewy limbs. May have eye anomalies, such as crossed eyes.

Key Clues: Well defined musculature and sinews even when not fit, hard to make their coats shine.

Feel to touch: Very firm to the point of being tense.

Motivating force: Challenge.

They value: Direction.

They hate: To be blocked.

Most likely to find them: Waiting by the door impatiently.

The Wood type likes to get things done and is motivated by challenge. Wood types are adventurous by nature and like to be the best. If their ambition or desire for action is thwarted they are impatient and can lash out, especially if they are tired. They dread confinement, and like the freedom to make choices and having a sense of purpose. They often enjoy competing and need to be given a goal in order to learn easily. They usually give the impression of having unending energy that never quite relaxes and are hard to keep up with. They can also be very stubborn as they have great confidence in doing things their own way.

Out of Balance they can get so goal-oriented they trip over their own feet. This causes them to get tense, which causes them to rush even more, until they collapse in a heap, jittery, bad-tempered and depressed. They are likely to suffer from liver or tendon problems, compulsive behaviour, depression and conditions that move around the body unpredictably.

In essence: They love action but can easily over do it, they are the competition star that suddenly breaks down becoming depressed and despondent. Or the animal that switches off because of boredom and a meaningless routine, often lashing out in frustration.

They need: A stimulating environment, flexibility, clear direction, patient handling. A simple, toxin-free diet.

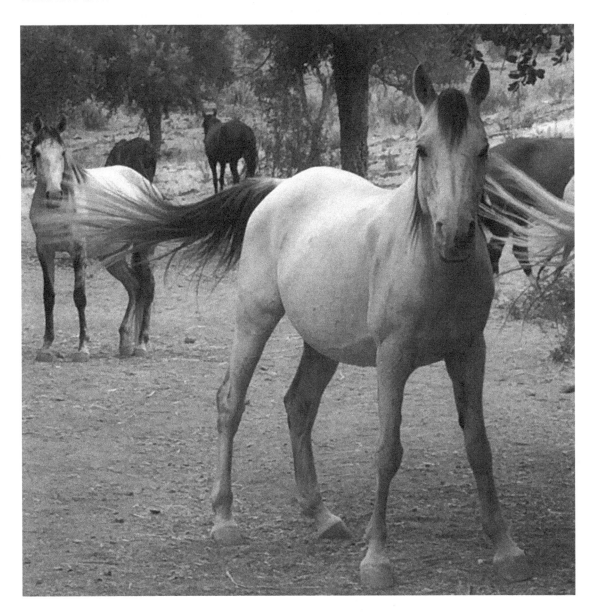

FIRE - THE ENTERTAINER

» The meridians: Heart/Small Intestine and Pericardium/Triple Warmer

» Season: Summer

» Climate: Heat

» Time of day: Midday

» Emotion: Joy

» Feeds Earth, controlled by Water, controls Metal

Physical Appearance: Willowy, graceful, long neck and limbs, soft warm pliant skin, fine coat, moves gracefully and lightly.

Key Clues: Elegant, light-boned, fine coat or mane and tail, attractive, playful.

Feel to touch: Warm and silky, you just want to stroke them.

Motivating Force: Connection.

They value: Warmth.

They hate: Isolation.

Most likely to find them: At the centre of attention.

The Fire type is intelligent, friendly, and demonstrative, looking for connection. They are charismatic and confident, attracting admiration and drawing others to them. They like excitement and emotional drama, and love being in the limelight. There is also the Heart Protector archetype who appears shy at first, only warming up after he is familiar with the person or surroundings.

Out of balance, this playful sense of the joy of life can become over-exaggerated and may become frenzied or over-agitated, even a sort of nervous hysteria. This state can often be triggered by being left alone. They can become oversensitive to stimuli, making them shy or timid, or alternatively, hysterical. Once their fire has burnt out they can become despondent, relying on others for their sense of identity. They are likely to suffer from hot conditions of the skin, arrhythmia, hyper-reactivity.

In essence: Fire types are the highly strung animals that are great fun to be around but can turn into a dithering wreck, shying/yapping over imaginary ghosts. Sometimes they seem to imagine the ghosts to entertain themselves.

They need: Calmness, physical affection and playfulness. A cooling diet, with added pro-biotics.

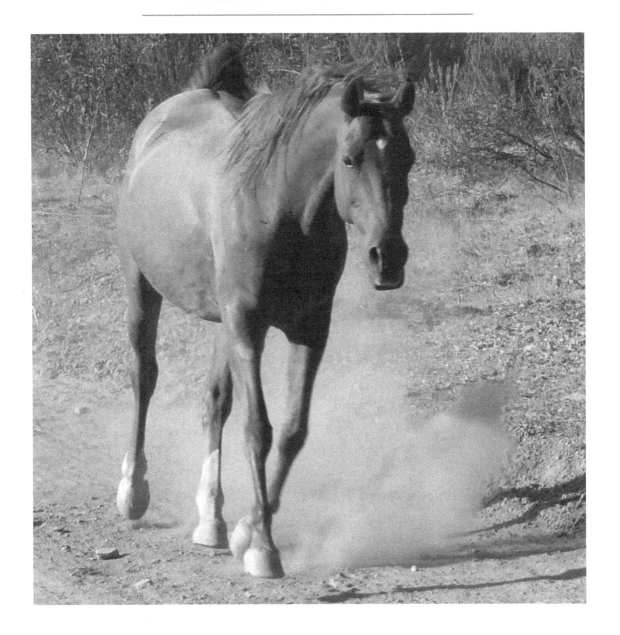

EARTH - THE PEACEMAKER

» The meridians: Spleen-Pancreas/Stomach

» Season: Late Summer

» Climate: Damp

» Time of day: Afternoon

» Emotion: Sympathy (Worry)

» Feeds Metal, controls Water, controlled by Wood

Physical appearance: Round physique, well muscled and broad, with a tendency to run to fat. Their feet may look small. They move rhythmically but heavily and their coats are often rather coarse.

Key Clues: Small feet for their size; round tummy and quarters; rather square, heavy head.

Feel to touch: Fleshy.

Motivating force: Harmony.

They value: Comfort.

They hate: Change and upsets in their world.

Most likely to find them: In the kitchen, figuratively and literally.

The Earth type is the mother of the world - although not necessarily female! - always caring for the needs of others before their own. They exude a calm and grounded aura, along with great endurance and a kind nature. They like routine, security and stability, and don't take kindly to changes. They like to feel needed, and are happiest if everyone is in the same place, moving harmoniously together.

Out of balance they can become over-concerned and anxious about the welfare of others, obsessing about everyone else and 'losing their mind' with worry; or they can be confused and lacking in focus. They can start feeling hard-done-by and unappreciated, demanding constant emotional validation, and will become apathetic if these emotional needs are not met. They are very food oriented, especially if they feel insecure, and have a tendency to put on weight. They are likely to suffer from Damp conditions such as fungal infections and wet excema.

In essence: Because they love being needed and having a fixed routine the typical Earth animal is happy when it knows what its role is and is appreciated for its efforts. For example, in the centre of a happy family with a regular routine, or as a riding school horse.

They need: Stability, to feel needed but not over-burdened with responsibility. It is very important to keep their weight down and feed a sugar-free diet. Earth dogs should be fed a grain-free diet.

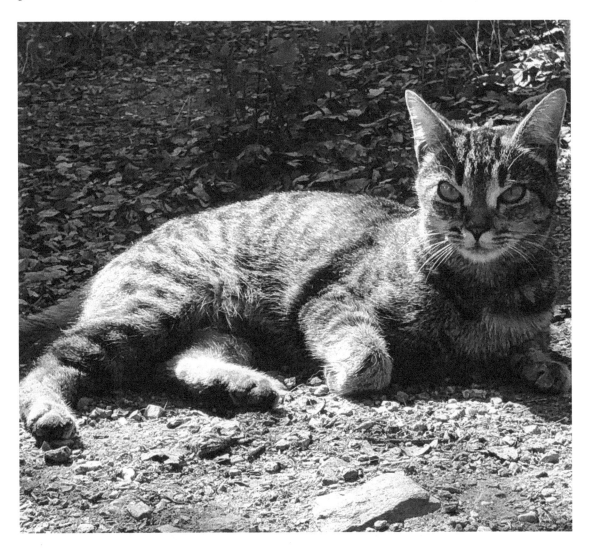

METAL - THE IDEALIST

- » The meridians: Lung/Large Intestine
- » Season: Autumn
- » Climate: Dryness
- » Time of day: Evening
- » Emotion: Grief
- » Feeds Water; controlled by Fire; controls Wood

Physical appearance: Neat, trim, slightly angular, with delicate features, small bones and compact muscles, moves in a tidy, economical fashion. Their coats have a tendency to be dry and brittle.

Key Clues: Angular; economical movement, polite, unassuming.

Feel to touch: Slightly prickly, dry.

Motivating force: Clarity.

They value: Clear communication.

They hate: Disorder.

Most likely to find them: Just behind the leader of the pack/herd.

The Metal Type loves order and has a well-defined, sometimes inflexible, sense of right and wrong. They can appear aloof, but enjoy learning and appreciate being treated as an equal partner. They are thoughtful animals who enjoy engaging their minds and appreciate consistency. They find it hard to forgive being reprimanded unfairly and are very sensitive to their environment, where they also like to feel a sense of orderliness and calm. They demand that others respect their boundaries and can be quite aggressive about imposing this. They have a great respect for authority and try to do what is asked, feeling very bad when told off. However the authority figure must meet the Metal types' exacting standards for fairness and clarity and show respect, or else Metal will feel confused and betrayed.

Out of Balance, if their need for order and correctness is not met, Metal types will withdraw into themselves becoming rigid and snappish. Or they may become completely subservient, as they lose touch with their instincts, no longer trust their own sense of right and wrong, and rely entirely on others to tell them what to do. They commonly suffer from asthma, allergies, irritable bowel syndrome or immune system disorders.

In essence: Metal types often make good teachers, but they can also be easily overlooked as they generally do not push themselves forward or make a fuss about life until it is intolerable for them. But if you are sensitive to early quiet complaints and don't feel insulted by their slightly stand-offish nature, you will find you have a stalwart partner.

They need: To be treated fairly and with respect and to know what the rules are; a structured learning environment; a clean, uncluttered environment.

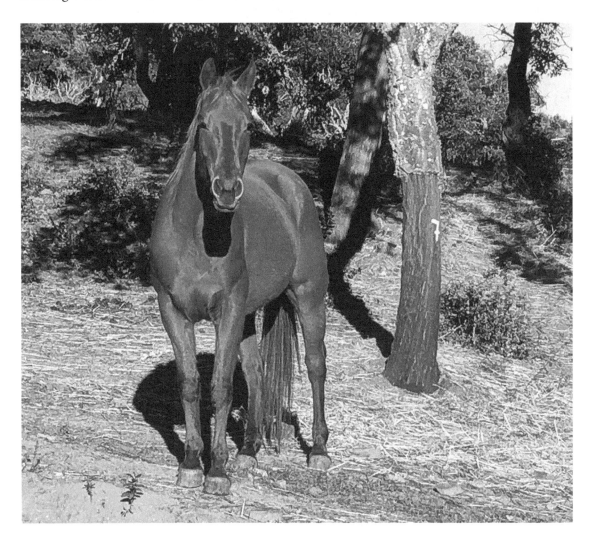

FIVE ELEMENT QUESTIONNAIRE

To figure out which element is predominant in your animal's character read the five answers to each question carefully, decide which answer is MOST TYPICAL of your animal and give it a mark of 5, mark the least likely response as 1, and the others 2, 3 and 4 in order of similarity to your animal. Each lettered question should be given a number.

Try to be objective about the answers and remember that you are choosing what is the most usual response. It is an interesting exercise for each member of the family to answer the quiz independently, as each point of view will reflect the element of the person answering (yes, that is a factor too).

When answering you must also take into account what is typical for the species, e.g. horses will instinctively want to run from something scary, but how does yours deal with that instinct? Age and breed will also affect the appearance of behaviour; however, your animal will have its own unique tendencies. Answer from your gut without thinking about it too hard and you will find it easier, if the questions are not things you have experienced firsthand then imagine the situation.

When you have completed the quiz, add up the points for each letter, (i.e. what is the total number of points for each A answer, each B answer, etc.) and see which letter has the highest points, then check which element that letter represents (letter key at the bottom of the page). The letter with the highest points is the primary element. If there is an element that has significantly less points than the others it indicates a deficiency, so you could also choose oils to strengthen the deficient element. This is a quiz in which there are no right or wrong answers, enjoy!

1. You and your animal go on an adventure, does he most typically:
   A. Relish the experience and come alive
   B. Get excited and nervous but has fun
   C. Get worried and anxious but as long as we're together....
   D. Assess the situation coolly and get on with it
   E. Would rather go home

2. You want to show off your animal's skills. When 'center stage', does she most typically:
   A. Enjoy the challenge and give it his best shot
   B. Revel in the limelight but get a bit goofy
   C. Mess up stuff she has been doing perfectly

D. Carry on regardless, carefully ignoring the attention

E. Refuse to participate

3. Your usual routine has changed, is your animal most typically:

A. Impatient and pushy

B. Really excited to see you, wants to play all the time

C. Anxious and demanding of your attention

D. A bit standoffish

E. Outwardly cool, but withdrawn, possibly restless

4. Your animal most typically learns best through:

A. Simple direction

B. Play

C. Repetition

D. Precise explanation

E. Figuring it out in his own time

5. When your animal is scared he will most typically:

A. Lash out

B. Fool around/get hysterical

C. Demand attention

D. Get guarded and spiky

E. Disappear

6. Would you describe your animal's approach to life as most typically:

A. Forward fast

B. Curious

C. Lazy

D. Considered

E. Cautious

7. When meeting a new person your animal is most likely to be:
    A. Quite forward, even a little intimidating
    B. Excited and curious, or shy
    C. Friendly and demonstrative
    D. Polite but distant
    E. Suspicious

8. When your animal is eating she will most typically:
    A. Keep one eye on the competition
    B. Always be ready to leave for something more interesting
    C. Forget anything else exists
    D. Pick and choose the best bits and leave the rest
    E. Eat because she must

9. The most important thing in your animal's life is:
    A. Action
    B. Playmates
    C. Harmony
    D. Personal space
    E. A quiet place to retreat to

10. Your animal least tolerates:
    A. Boredom
    B. Isolation
    C. Conflict
    D. Confusion
    E. Noise

11. Which of these best describes your animal?

    A. The Organiser

    B. The Playmate

    C. The Sympathiser

    D. The Observer

    E. The Philosopher

12. How does your animal like to be touched?

    A. A good solid pat or massage as a sign of solidarity

    B. Soft caresses

    C. Can't get enough hugs and attention

    D. Doesn't really like to be touched except by a few special people

    E. Will come to you for a cuddle in his own good time

Codes: A=Wood/ B=Fire / C= Earth / D=Metal / E= Water

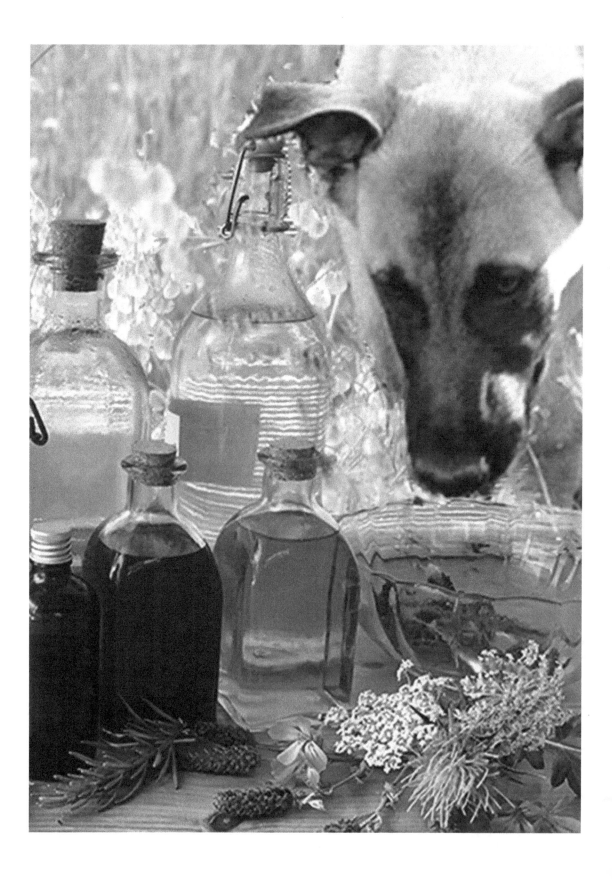

CHAPTER 4

MATERIA AROMATICA

The Materia Aromatica contains all the information you need to choose the best essential oil, hydrosol and carrier oil for your animal.

1. Essential oil /hydrosol cross reference chart (MA1)

Find which essential oil or hydrosol best matches the physical and emotional picture of your animal and his problem.

2. Index of Essential oils for specific conditions (MA2)

A comprehensive listing of health and behaviour problems and the essential oils/hydrosols that can help.

3. Essential oil profiles (MA3)

Detailed description of 56 essential oils and their uses

4. Carrier Oil profiles (MA4)

Detailed description of 12 vegetable and macerated herbal oils, and their uses

5. Hydrosol profiles (MA5)

Descriptions of 24 hydrosols, what they do and when to use them.

6. Index of essential oils & hydrosols for specific meridians (MA6)

A listing of which essential oils are best suited to specific meridian systems.

7. Index of Therapeutic Actions (MA7)

Find which essential oil is anti-inflammatory, analgesic, etc.

ESSENTIAL OIL/HYDROSOL CROSS REFERENCE CHART (MA1)

ESSENTIAL OIL	ELEMENT	PHYSICAL INDICATORS	EMOTIONAL INDICATORS	COMMON USES	KEYWORD	CAUTIONS
Angelica root *Angelica archangelica*	Water (Earth, Fire)	Heart disturbances, sluggish digestion, loss of appetite, hepatitis, fungal infection, immune problems, shortness of breath.	Hysteria, 'switched off', nervous, fearful, hyperactive.	For animals who are closed to healing, early-life trauma, fearful reactivity, debilitation, multiple problems.	**Healing angel**	Photo toxic.
Basil, French *Ocimum basilicum*	Metal (Earth)	Muscle pain, lung congestion, nerve tremors, indigestion, flatulence.	Distracted, lack of concentration.	Muscle pain, distracted, flighty animals, nervous exhaustion, strangles.	**Think!**	Possible sensitizer, dilute well.
Benzoin *Benzoin styrax*	Earth (Metal)	Cracked skin, scars, skeletal weakness, relieves coughs, releases trauma.	Angry fear, worry and over-thinking, withdrawn when anxious, stoic.	Past trauma especially around physical scars, cracked feet, weak back.	**Strengthen**	Possible sensitizer, dilute well.
Bergamot *Citrus aurantium, subsp, bergamia*	Wood (Fire, Water)	Tumours and growths, warts, sarcoids, bacterial infection of lungs or urinary tract, hormone imbalance, viral infection.	Depression, mood swings.	Warts/tumours, infections of lungs or genito-urinary tract, balances emotions, post-parturition.	**Balancing**	Photo-toxic.
Cajeput *Melaleuca cajeputi Powell*	Metal	Bronchitis, chronic coughs, immune stimulant, strains, sprains, tight muscles.	Obsessive compulsion.	Arthritis, lung infections, compulsive habits.	**Clears**	Dilute well.
Carrotseed *Daucus carota*	Wood & Earth	Poor skin/hooves, liver, underweight, heart problems, cuts and bruises, smooth muscle relaxant.	Despair, abandonment.	Malnutrition, feet and coat, slow healing wounds, abandonment, haemorrhage.	**Regenerate**	Possible skin irritant.
Cedarwood Atlas *Cedrus atlantica*	Water (Metal)	Coughs with white mucous, skin infections, insect repellent, general tonic, kidney problems, poor circulation, hair loss.	Insecurity, timorous, ungrounded.	Lymphatic drainage, coughs, backache, oedema, genito-urinary, timidity.	**Stabilizing**	
Chamomile German *Matricaria recutita*	Wood & Earth	Swellings, allergies, fungal infections, stomach upsets, itchy skin.	Anxiety, irritability, stress manifesting in the body.	Itchy skin, allergies, inflammation, fungal infections.	**Anti-irritant**	
Chamomile Roman *Anthemis nobilis*	Wood (Earth)	Nervous stomach, irritable skin, red eyes, runny eyes.	Highly strung, nervousness, tantrums.	General nervousness, skin irritation, angry outbursts, nervous upset stomach, problems with children.	**The Child**	Possible sensitisation.

ESSENTIAL OIL	ELEMENT	PHYSICAL INDICATORS	EMOTIONAL INDICATORS	COMMON USES	KEYWORD	CAUTIONS
Chastetree *Vitex Agnus Castus*	Earth (Fire)	Metabolic syndrome, endocrine dysfunction, hormonal imbalance	Sluggish, nervous, intolerant, despairing, bad-tempered	Irregular cycles, Cushing's, Addison's, enlarged prostate, metabolic syndrome		
Cistus/Rock rose *Cistus ladaniferus*	Metal	Damaged skin, itching, bruises, scars, circulation, Immune modulator	Detached, fearful, over-reactive, blocked emotions	Itchy skin, scar healing, emotional detachment, any skin condition	**Regenerate**	
Clary Sage *Salvia sclarea*	Metal (Earth)	Tight muscles, respiratory distress, dry skin, hormonal imbalance.	Fearful, hyper-reactive, tense.	Asthma, muscle spasm, hormonal imbalance, tension, fear.	**Relaxing**	Do not use with alchohol.
Cypress *Cupressus sempervirens*	Metal (Water)	Thyroid problems, genito-urinary problems, excess fluids, sluggish circulation.	Grieving, withdrawn, insecure.	Grief, asthma, change of circumstances, excess or deficient perspiration	**Let-go**	
Elemi *Canarium luzonicum*	Metal (Fire)	Dry skin, tight breathing, immune deficiency.	Scattered, 'all over the place', no inner peace, erratic.	Old skin, immune, asthma, balancing both sides of body.	**Harmonize**	
Eucalyptus *Globulus/Radiata*	Metal	Upper respiratory congestion, chronic nasal dampness, muscle pain, fungal infections.	Claustrophobia, frustration.	Fever, congestions of the respiratory tract, thrush, insect repellent, sinusitis	**Disinfect**	Oral toxin.
Fennel *Foeniculum vulgare var., dulce.*	Earth	Flatulence, fatty lumps, lack/excess of milk, indigestion, excess hormones, poisoning.	Worry, over-concerned about others, emotionally needy.	False pregnancy, lactation problems, stomach upset, fluid retention, flatulence, obesity.	**Reassuring**	Avoid in pregnancy.
Flouve *Anthoxanthum odoratum*	Metal (Wood)	Anti-allergenic, anti-tumour, immune stimulant.	Slight irritability and space protective.	Allergies, run-down animals, tumours.	**Like cures like**	Do not use with blood thinning drugs.
Frankincense *Boswellia carterii*	Earth (Metal)	Shortness of breath, nervous digestive upsets, dry, flaky skin, scars, skin ulcers, tumours	Nervous fear, specific fears, worry, anxiety	Box walking, diarrhoea, asthma, nervous cough, break with past, fear of known things, fireworks.	**Distances**	
Garlic *Allium sativum*	Metal (Earth, Fire)	Lung infections, heart congestion, bacterial infection.	Weak, sluggish, inhibited, forlorn.	Bacterial infections of all kind, heart problems, insect infestation.	**Antibiotic**	Harsh on skin.

ESSENTIAL OIL	ELEMENT	PHYSICAL INDICATORS	EMOTIONAL INDICATORS	COMMON USES	KEYWORD	CAUTIONS
Geranium *Pelargonium graveolens*	Water (Fire)	Hormonal, dandruff, endocrine imbalance, sluggish liver/kidneys.	Mood swings, overwhelmed insecure.	Hormonal problems, insecurity, new home, dry skin, lice.	**Regulates**	Possible sensitizer.
Ginger *Zingiber officinale*	Fire (Water, Earth)	Arthritis, older animals, muscle stiffness, sore back, lung congestion, respiratory infection, digestive.	Depression, self-protective, overwhelmed by life, no self-confidence.	Sluggish systems and overall weakness, excess damp conditions, lack of willpower.	**Stimulating**	Slightly harsh on skin.
Grapefruit *Citrus x paradisi*	Wood	Run-down, overweight, bad breath, lymphatic congestion.	Mild depression, lack of zest.	Sluggish systems, lymphatic drainage, detox, lethargy, obesity.	**Refreshes**	Slight photo-toxicity.
Hay SEE FLOUVE						
Helichrysum *Helichrysum italicum*	Wood (Metal)	Traumatic injury, allergies, run-down, multiple problems, congestion, bruising, tendon injuries.	Deep emotional wounds that linger.	Bruises, damaged tissue, past trauma, allergic skin conditions.	**Tender care**	
Hemp *Cannabis sativa, L*	Wood (Fire)	Tight muscles, high blood pressure, eye problems.	Hyper-sensitive, insecure, depressed, aggressive.	Aggression, fear, hyperactivity, nausea, muscle tightness.	**Motivator**	
Hyssop *Hysopus officinalis var decumbens*	Metal	Dry coughs, stomach bloat, sluggishness.	Prone to 'falling apart', oversensitive to the moods of others.	Defensive aggression, general tonic, over-reactivity, general weakness.	**The Protector**	
Jasmine *Jasminum officinale*	Fire (Water)	Male hormone balancer, mildly analgesic.	Nervous anxiety, over 'Yang' behaviour, insecure pushiness.	Pushy, bullying behaviour, hierarchy issues, anxiety, sexual anxiety.	**Chill out**	
Juniperberry *Juniperis communis*	Water (Metal, Wood)	Arthritis, muscle strain, soft tissue damage, weak kidneys, sluggish systems.	Disturbed mind, unsettled, aloof, gloomy, worried about themselves.	Arthritis, after hard work, post-op, soft tissue damage, clearing mind.	**Cleanses**	Overuse can damage kidneys.
Lavender *Lavandula angustifolia*	Fire (Earth)	Accident prone, sensitive skin, heart palpitations.	Restless anxiety, mood swings, shyness.	Wounds, burns, proud flesh, sweet itch, mud fever, scars, hysteria.	**Florence Nightingale.**	Can cause tachycardia.
Lavender, Green *Lavandula viridis*	Earth (Metal)	Opens lungs, clears sinus, anti-fungal, heals skin	Exhausted from caring, sad, lonely, needs support	Fungal infections, respiratory infection, depressed and rundown	**Community carer**	Caution with children

ESSENTIAL OIL	ELEMENT	PHYSICAL INDICATORS	EMOTIONAL INDICATORS	COMMON USES	KEYWORD	CAUTIONS
Lemon *Citrus limon*	Earth (Fire, Water)	Run-down, sluggish liver and kidney, arthritis, ringbone, immune problems.	Slight depression, lack of trust in self or others, confusion, lack of focus.	Kidney stones, bony growths, immune disease, run down, kidney disease.	Pick me up	
Lemongrass *Cymbopogon citratus*	Earth	Compromised immune system, growths, muscle pain, arthritis.	Emotionally needy, unfocused, insecure, worried.	Fly/flea repellent, tumours, depression, confusion, pain.	**Dissolves**	Possible skin sensitisation, dilute well.
Lentisk *Pistacia lentiscus*	Metal	Stiffness, gum infections, tumours and growths	Hard to connect, unsettled, seems wild	Dental care, skin growths, arthritis. Immune support. When its hard to connect	**Liberates**	
Manuka *Leptospermum scoparium*	Metal	Skin problems, allergies, wounds, nervous respiratory disorders and lung infections.	Withdrawn, self-protective.	Bacterial infection, skin problems, colds and flu.	**Skin heal**	
Marjoram, sweet. *Origanum majorana*	Earth.	Lowers blood pressure, cleansing, nervous tension, reduces sexual drive.	Grief, hyperactivity, "no-one cares".	Bereavement, sore muscles, strengthens nerves, worry/anxiety over others, ticks.	**Nurturing**	Avoid with low blood pressure.
Melissa (Lemon Balm) *Melissa officinalis*	Fire & Wood	Poor immune system, allergies, viral infection, herpes, sluggish digestion, hormonal irregularity.	Hyperactive, over-reactive, nervous, jittery, forlorn, over-sensitive.	Herpes, respiratory infections, viruses, warts, auto-immune disease, hyperactivity, no trust.	**Fast relief**	Do not use with glaucoma.
Myrrh *Commiphora myrrha*	Earth (Metal)	Oozing skin conditions, chronic coughs, diarrhoea.	Overwhelmed with care, aloof, restless.	Fungal infections, weeping skin, persistent wet cough, mud-fever, hotspots.	**Desert wind**	Avoid in pregnancy.
Neroli (Orange blossom) *Citrus aurantium*	Fire (Wood)	Antidepressant, circulatory and heart tonic, hepatic, digestive.	Sadness, anxiety, loss of will to live.	Loss of companion, despondency, shock, stress-related colic, sadness of heart.	**Uplifting**	
Nutmeg *Myristica fragrans*	Earth (Fire)	Tight muscles, digestive upsets, loss of libido.	Needy, over-excitable.	Emotionally needy, nausea, flatulence, aches and pains.	**Attention seekers**	Dilute well.
Orange, sweet *Citrus sinensis*	Wood	Indigestion, juvenile colic, mouth ulcers.	Nervousness, depression.	Nervous tension especially in youngsters, obesity.	**Cheer up!**	

ESSENTIAL OIL	ELEMENT	PHYSICAL INDICATORS	EMOTIONAL INDICATORS	COMMON USES	KEYWORD	CAUTIONS
Patchouli *Pogostomen cablin*	Earth	Wet excema, mud fever, fungal infections, soft swellings, run down	Nervous exhaustion, stoic, long-suffering, bad-tempered.	Back pain, crusty skin eruptions, fly repellent, overheating, rain scald	**Chill out!**	
Peppermint *Mentha piperita*	Earth (Wood & Metal)	Nerve damage, indigestion, circulation, bruises, lung congestion, tendon strain.	Spaced out, 'knows best', lack of focus, defensive of personal space, snappy.	Lung congestion, sprains, colitis, colic, box rest, defensive aggression.	**Stimulates.**	Dilute well for topical use.
Plai *Zingiber cassumunar*	Water	Chronic pain, acute pain, tendon damage, nerve damage, digestive cramps.	Hothead, fearful anger, apathy, stubborn.	Pain, soft tissue damage, asthma, colic, boney growths, irritable bowel.	**Relieves**	
Ravensara *Ravensara aromatica*	Metal	Compromised immune, lung infections, run down.	Overwhelmed by life, 'spineless'.	Viral infection, herpes, neuro-muscular problems.	**Immune stimulant**	
Rhododendron *R. anthopogon*	Fire (Metal)	Metabolic imbalance, respiratory infection, tight muscles, adrenal exhaustion	Nervous, anxious, unsettled	Metabolic syndrome, extreme over-reactivity, bronchitis	**Adrenal tonic**	
Rosalina *Melaleuca ericifolia*	Metal	Skin and lung infections, convulsions.	Fretful.	Wounds, skin disorders, coughs/colds, thrush, infections.	**Gently cleanses**	
Rose *Rosa damascena*	Fire (Wood)	Hormonal problems, loss of appetite.	Past abuse, resentful, 'marish', self hate.	Female hormone problems, past abuse, depression.	**Self love**	Caution in pregnancy.
Rosemary *Rosmarinus officinalis*	Fire (Wood, Earth)	Muscle pain, general sluggishness, clumsiness, poor coat,	Hard to connect with, self-critical, no sense of self.	Alopecia, convalescence, muscle strain, sinus/lung congestion, lack of concentration.	**Brain power**	Avoid in pregnancy and epilepsy.
Spearmint *Mentha spicata*	Earth	Youngsters who have pain, digestive upsets, chronic pain, chronic dry cough.	Over-sensitive, troubled by life.	Digestive disorders with flatulence, respiratory mucous, muscle spasms.	**Delicate souls**	
Tansy *Tanacetum Anuum*	Wood (Metal)	Allergies, itchy skin, inflammation, head shaking	Irritable, withdrawn, disinterested	Allergic reactions in skin or lungs. Insect bites	**Anti-histamine**	Avoid use in pregnancy
Tea tree *Melaleuca alternifolia*	Metal	Run down, prone to infections.	Withdrawn, surly, stiff.	Infections of any kind, Immune stimulation.	**1st aid**	Cats, don't use. Dogs, dilute well.
Thyme *Thymus vulgaris*	Metal (Water)	Respiratory disease, bacterial infections, cold and trembling, food issues.	Fearful to the point of trembling, lethargic, withdrawn.	Fear, infections of lung, loose digestion, stagnation, lethargy.	**The brave oil.**	Dermal irritant, dilute well.

ESSENTIAL OIL	ELEMENT	PHYSICAL INDICATORS	EMOTIONAL INDICATORS	COMMON USES	KEYWORD	CAUTIONS
Valerian root *Valeriana officinalis*	Water	High blood pressure, nervous stomach, cramping pains.	Hysterical. Losing the mind through fear.	Panic, fear, restlessness, acute pain.	**Sedates**	Use in moderation.
Vanilla *Vanilla planifolia*	Earth	Soothing for emotions and stomach.	Irritable, moody, bitter.	Bad-tempered mares or bitches, irritability.	**Sweetens**	
Vetiver *Vetiveria zizanoides*	Earth (Water)	Under or overweight, poor doers, general stiffness and discomfort, anaemia.	Flighty, clumsy, bargy, over-excitable, clumsy, knocks into you.	Over excitability, 'no sense of their feet', weak constitution, debility.	**Grounding**	
Violet Leaf *Viola odorata*	Wood (Water)	Older animals with chronic pain, animals who move home or don't feel at home, congestive heart conditions.	Untrusting, flighty, spooky.	Loss of trust, new home, aches & pains, old grumps.	**Heart ease**	
Yarrow *Achillea millefolium*	Wood (Metal, Water)	Injuries of all types, self harm, allergies, irritated skin, liver or kidney congestion.	Past trauma, fearful anger, past abuse, unknown history.	Emotional/physical trauma, inflammation, itchy skin, wounds, allergies, insect bites.	**Releases**	Not to be used in pregnancy
Ylang-ylang *Cananga odorata*	Fire	High blood pressure, loss of libido, sensitive skin, hair loss.	Nervous, insecure, no self-confidence, no joi-de-vivre.	Hierarchy issues in young animals, dry skin, nervous exciteability,	**The Young Prince**	

ESSENTIAL OILS FOR SPECIFIC CONDITIONS (MA2)

This chart lists common health and behaviour problems and the essential oils, hydrosols and carrier oils that can help. It is organised by the anatomical system as in musculo-skeletal, digestive, etc. Cross reference with the other charts to match the oil to your animal's character for the most effective result.

CONDITION	ESSENTIAL OIL/ HYDROSOL	CARRIER OIL
CIRCULATION, MUSCLES, JOINTS		
Aches and Pains	Basil, benzoin, cajeput, carrot seed, cedarwood, cypress, clary sage, chamomile (both), ginger, helichrysum, juniper berry, lemongrass, lentisk, marjoram, nutmeg, peppermint, plai, rosemary, violet leaf, yarrow	Calendula, comfrey, hemp, hypericum, olive, sesame
Arthritis	Angelica root, basil, benzoin, cajeput, carrot seed, cedarwood, chamomile (German), fennel, ginger, hyssop, juniper berry, plai, seaweed, violet leaf, yarrow	Comfrey, hemp, hypericum, neem
Bony growths	Helichrysum, lemon, plai, violet leaf	Comfrey
Bruising	Cypress, chamomile, cistus, helichrysum, lavender, witch hazel	Comfrey, calendula, sunflower
Bursitis	Angelica root, cedarwood, cypress, grapefruit, helichrysum, juniper berry, yarrow	Comfrey, sunflower, calendula, neem
Cold (suffers from)	Benzoin, hemp, lentisk, marjoram, ginger, thyme	Hemp, hypericum
Circulation, stimulates	Basil, cajeput, clary sage, cedarwood, cypress, eucalyptus, ginger, lemongrass, peppermint, plai, rosemary, spearmint, thyme, vetiver	Hemp, hypericum
Capillaries/veins, broken	Cistu, cypress, carrot seed, chamomile, clary sage, helichrysum, lavender, rose	Comfrey, calendula, sunflower
Fluid retention	Angelica root, benzoin, cedarwood, chamomile, cypress, juniper berry, fennel (sweet), grapefruit	Hemp, hypericum, sunflower
Heart palpitations	Angelica root, benzoin, chamomile, marjoram, geranium, neroli, orange, rose, ylang-ylang	Calendula, hemp, sunflower, passionflower
Hypertension (high blood pressure)	Clary sage, garlic, lavender, marjoram (sweet), neroli, ylang-ylang	Calendula, olive hemp, passionflower, sunflower
Hypotension (low blood pressure)	Basil, cajeput, ginger, neroli, peppermint, rosemary, thyme, violet leaf	Olive, passionflower, sunflower,
Laminitis	Angelica root, basil, carrot seed, chamomile (German), garlic, neroli, patchouli, seaweed, violet leaf, yarrow	Calendula, sunflower, hemp, hypericum, grapeseed

Muscle cramps	Basil, clary sage, cypress, juniper berry, marjoram (sweet), seaweed, spearmint, yarrow	Hemp, sunflower, calendula
Muscle fatigue	Basil, grapefruit, juniper berry, lemongrass, lentisk, peppermint, rosemary, spearmint, thyme	Hemp, sunflower, calendula
Muscle strain	Chamomile, clary sage, helichrysum, marjoram (sweet), nutmeg, peppermint, plai, yarrow, rhododendron	Calendula, hemp, hypericum, sunflower
Muscle stiffness	Basil, cedarwood, clary sage, eucalyptus, ginger, juniper berry, lemongrass, marjoram, nutmeg, plai	Comfrey, hemp, hypericum, olive, sesame
Navicular	Angelica root, benzoin, cajeput, garlic, lemon, lemongrass, peppermint, plai, rosemary, seaweed, violet leaf, yarrow	Comfrey, calendula, neem, sunflower
Neuro-muscular problems	Angelica root, basil, cajeput, chamomile (Roman), lentisk, peppermint, plai, ravensara, rhododendron	Calendula, hypericum, sunflower
Oedema	Angelica root, basil, cedarwood, cypress, helichrysum, juniper berry, lime, lemon, lentisk, nutmeg, peppermint, rosemary, thyme	Sunflower, comfrey, calendula
Tendon damage	Chamomile (German), cajeput, helichrysum, juniper berry, lavender, peppermint, plai, spearmint, ravensara, yarrow	Comfrey, calendula, neem, sunflower

DIGESTIVE SYSTEM

Anorexia/loss of appetite	Angelica root, benzoin, bergamot, carrot seed, ginger, hyssop, peppermint	Hemp, olive, sesame, sunflower
Bloating	Basil, carrot seed, chamomile (Roman), fennel (sweet), grapefruit, hyssop, peppermint, plai	Calendula, olive, sesame, sunflower
Colic	Angelica root, basil, carrot seed, chamomile, fennel (sweet), lemongrass, marjoram (sweet), neroli, orange (sweet), peppermint, plai, spearmint	Olive, sunflower
Colitis	Carrot seed, chamomile, grapefruit, lentisk, peppermint, plai, spearmint	Calendula, olive grapeseed, sunflower, sesame
Constipation	Basil, fennel (sweet), ginger, orange (sweet), peppermint, seaweed	Olive, sunflower
Diarrhoea	Benzoin, Roman chamomile, frankincense, ginger, lentisk, myrrh, neroli, thyme, rhododendron	Calendula, grapeseed, sesame
Digestive disturbances	Angelica root, chamomile, grapefruit (chronic), fennel (sweet), frankincense, neroli, orange, peppermint, spearmint, thyme, vanilla	Calendula, hemp, grapeseed, olive, sunflower
Flatulence	Basil, bergamot, fennel (sweet), ginger, spearmint, chastetree	Hemp, olive, sunflower

Food obsessed	Basil, bergamot, fennel, grapefruit	Sunflower, grapeseed, olive
Irritable bowel syndrome	Carrot seed, chamomile, grapefruit, lentisk, marjoram, peppermint, plai, spearmint	Hemp, olive, sunflower
Liver deficiency	Angelica root, carrot seed, geranium, grapefruit, helichrysum, juniper berry, lemon, lime, seaweed	Calendula, sunflower, olive
Malnutrition (past and present),	Carrot seed, lemon, seaweed, vetiver	Hemp, olive, sunflower
Mouth ulcers	Benzoin, bergamot, frankincense, lentisk, myrrh, rosalina, orange (sweet), tea tree, thyme	Sunflower, grapeseed, aloe vera gel
Nausea	Basil, chamomile, ginger, peppermint, plai, spearmint	Hemp, sunflower, grapeseed, olive
Obesity	Basil, cedarwood, fennel, grapefruit, orange (sweet), chastetree	Grapeseed, sunflower, olive
Pancreatic Problems	Angelica root, chamomile (German), cedarwood, fennel, ginger, seaweed, chastetree	Calendula, comfrey, olive, sesame
Sluggish Digestion	Basil, fennel, ginger, grapefruit, nutmeg, plai, thyme	Grapeseed, hemp, sunflower, olive
Stress-related digestive problems	Angelica root, benzoin, chamomile, frankincense, neroli	Grapeseed, hemp, olive, passion flower, sesame, sunflower
Worms	Bergamot, cajeput, carrot seed, garlic, hyssop, plai, thyme	Hemp, olive, sunflower
Ulcers	Angelica root, benzoin, chamomile (German), frankincense, lentisk	Calendula, comfrey, sunflower
Underweight	Angelica root, benzoin, lemon, seaweed, vetiver	Hemp, olive, sesame, sunflower

IMMUNE SYSTEM

Allergies	Basil, cistus, chamomile (German), flouve, helichrysum, tansy, yarrow, rhododendron	Calendula, hemp, neem, olive, passionflower, sesame
Anaemia	Carrot seed, chamomile (Roman), seaweed, vetiver	Hemp, olive, sesame
Auto immune diseases	Angelica root, bergamot, carrot seed, chamomile, flouve, grapefruit, juniper berry, lemon, melissa, seaweed, rhododendron	Grapeseed, hemp, hypericum, olive, sunflower
Bacterial infections	Basil, bergamot, eucalyptus, ginger, helichrysum, lavender white, manuka (staphylococcus & other gram-positive infections), thyme, tea tree	Calendula, comfrey, hypericum, olive
Fever	Basil, bergamot, cajeput, eucalyptus, lavender white, rosalina	Calendula, grapeseed, sunflower

Immune deficiency	Angelica root, bergamot, cajeput, chamomile, eucalyptus, flouve, hyssop, lemon, lime, manuka, patchouli, ravensara, seaweed, tea tree, vetiver	Grapeseed, hemp, olive, sesame, sunflower
Influenza	Angelica root, basil, benzoin, cajeput, eucalyptus, ginger, grapefruit, lavender, lavender white, lemon, lime, manuka, ravensara, rosalina, rosemary, tea tree, thyme, rhododendron	Carrot, hemp, olive, sesame
Lethargy	Cedarwood, lemon, lentisk, lime, peppermint, orange, rosemary, thyme, chastetree	Hemp, sesame, Passionflower
Tumours	Bergamot, cistus, fennel (sweet), flouve, frankincense, hay, lentisk, seaweed	Carrot, comfrey, hemp, sunflower
Viral infections	Basil, bergamot, eucalyptus, helichrysum, hyssop, lemon, lavender, lavender white, marjoram, peppermint, ravensara, rosemary, tea tree	Grapeseed, hemp, neem, olive, sesame, sunflower

NERVOUS SYSTEM

Head shaking	Basil, cajeput, flouve, hay, lemon, peppermint, rosemary, tansy	Sunflower, hypericum
Nerve damage	Basil, peppermint	Hypericum
Nerve tonic	Angelica root, basil, cedarwood, cistus, clary sage, lemongrass, neroli	Hypericum, passionflower, sunflower
Nervous exhaustion	Angelica root, basil, benzoin, chamomile (Roman), clary sage, helichrysum, hemp, lavender white, lemon, vanilla	hemp, hypericum. passionflower, sunflower
Wobbler syndrome	juniper berry, lemon, peppermint, plai, rosemary	Hypericum, olive, sunflower,
Epilepsy	Clary sage, rosemary hydrosol, marjoram	Sunflower, hypericum

REPRODUCTIVE AND ENDOCRINE SYSTEM

Addison's	Angelica root, geranium, lemon, frankincense, peppermint, seaweed, chastetree	Hemp, grapeseed, passionflower
Cushing's disease	Angelica root, flouve, geranium, peppermint, seaweed, chastetree	Hemp, grapeseed, passionflower
Irregular cycle	Sweet fennel, chamomile, geranium, rose, yarrow, chastetree	Hemp, hypericum, sunflower
Genital infections	Bergamot, clary sage, chamomile, lavender,	Calendula, grapeseed, hypericum
Hormonal problems	Bergamot, chamomile (german), clary sage, cypress, geranium, jasmine, sweet fennel, rose, yarrow, chastetree	Hemp, hypericum, olive, sunflower
Hypothyroidism	Cypress, geranium, seaweed, chastetree	Grapeseed, olive, sunflower
Insufficient milk	Basil, fennel (sweet)	Comfrey, hypericum

Libido (too little)	Cedarwood, jasmine, ylang-ylang, ginger	Grapeseed, olive, passionflower, sunflower
Libido (too much)	Marjoram (sweet), hemp, jasmine, ylang-ylang	Hemp, grapeseed, olive, sunflower
Metabolic syndrome	Angelica root, bergamot, carrot seed, cypress, geranium, peppermint, rose, seaweed, chastetree, rhododendron	Hemp, hypericum, grapeseed, olive, sunflower
Moody mares	Bergamot, clary sage, cypress, geranium, jasmine, sweet fennel, rose, vanilla, chastetree, rhododendron	Calendula, hemp, hypericum, sunflower
Phantom pregnancy	Clary Sage, sweet fennel, geranium, hemp, lavender white, peppermint, rose, vetiver, yarrow, chastetree	Calendula, hypericum, grapeseed, olive, sunflower
Post parturition	Bergamot, chamomile (both), sweet fennel, jasmine, rose, yarrow	Calendula, olive, sunflower
Uncomfortable heat/ season	Cypress, clary sage, chamomile, marjoram, rose yarrow, chastetree	Calendula, hemp, hypericum, olive

RESPIRATORY SYSTEM

Airborne bacteria (kills)	Bergamot, eucalyptus, garlic, thyme	Do not dilute in oil
Allergies	Chamomile (German), flouve, hay, helichrysum, spearmint, tansy, yarrow, rhododendron	Calendula, comfrey, hemp
Asthma	Benzoin, cedarwood, clary sage, cypress, elemi, eucalyptus, hyssop, frankincense, helichrysum, peppermint, plai, rhododendron	Comfrey, hemp, sunflower
Bronchitis	Angelica root, basil, benzoin, cajeput, eucalyptus, garlic, ginger, helichrysum, lavaender white, peppermint, thyme, tea tree, rhododendron	Comfrey, hemp, olive, sunflower
Excess mucous	Angelica root, benzoin, cedarwood, lavender white, myrrh, spearmint, peppermint, thyme, rhododendron	Comfrey, hemp, olive, sunflower
Exercise-induced pulmonary haemorrhage	Carrot seed, helichrysum, yarrow	Carrot, comfrey, hemp, sunflower
Infections (general respiratory)	Angelica root, basil, benzoin, cajeput, garlic, hyssop, lavender white, ravensara, rosalina, tea tree, thyme, rhododendron	Carrot, comfrey, hemp, olive, sunflower
Influenza	Angelica root, basil, benzoin, cajeput, eucalyptus, ginger, grapefruit, lavender, lavender white, lemon, lime, manuka, ravensara, rosalina, rosemary, tea tree, thyme, rhododendron	Carrot, comfrey, hemp, olive, sunflower
Kennel cough	Angelica root, basil, bergamot, cajeput, eucalyptus, lavender white, lemon, garlic, manuka, peppermint, rosalina, rosemary, tea tree, thyme, rhododendron	Carrot, comfrey, hemp, olive, sunflower

Pneumonitis	Garlic, eucalyptus, lavender white, manuka, rosalina, tea tree, thyme	Comfrey, olive, sunflower
Recurrent airway obstruction (RAO, COPD)	Eucalyptus, clary sage, flouve, frankincense, hay, helichrysum, myrrh, peppermint, tansy, rhododendron	Carrot, comfrey, hemp, olive, sunflower
Sinus problems	Benzoin, cajeput, eucalyptus, flouve, ginger, hay, lavender, lavender white, peppermint, rosemary, rhododendron	Calendula, grapeseed, hemp, sunflower
Strangles	Basil, benzoin, bergamot, cajeput, eucalyptus, garlic, ginger, lavender white, manuka, rosalina, rosemary, tea tree, thyme, rhododendron	Carrot, comfrey, hemp, olive, sunflower

SKIN (INCLUDING HOOF AND NAILS)

Allergic dermatitis	Bergamot, chamomile (German), cistus, helichrysum, Tansy	Calendula, hemp, sunflower
Alopecia (hair loss)	Carrot seed, cedarwood, chamomile (Roman), clary sage, rosemary, ylang-ylang	Carrot, hemp, olive, sunflower
Anhidrosis (lack of sweating)	Angelica root, basil (sweet), bergamot, cajeput, cypress, rosalina, spearmint, seaweed, tea tree	Comfrey, calendula, hemp, olive, sesame
Coat (poor)	Carrot seed, seaweed	Carrot, hemp, olive, sesame
Eczema	Cistus, chamomile, helichrysum, lavender, yarrow	Calendula, hemp, neem, sunflower
Fungal infections	Angelica root, bergamot, cedarwood, clary sage, chamomile (German), fennel, geranium, helichrysum, lavender, lavender white, lentisk, lemon, lemongrass, manuka, myrrh, patchouli, rosemary, tea tree	Carrot, calendula, neem, olive
Flea/ Fly repellent	Basil, cajeput, cedarwood, cistus, cypress, eucalyptus, garlic, geranium, lavender, lemongrass, manuka, patchouli, peppermint, tansy, vetiver	Neem, sunflower, grapeseed
Granulomas	Cistus, chamomile (German), geranium, lavender, manuka, myrrh, rosalina, yarrow	Calendula, comfrey, hypericum, neem
Hoof abscesses	Carrot seed, garlic, lavender white, manuka, seaweed, tea tree, thyme	Carrot, comfrey, sunflower
Hooves (poor)	Carrot seed, garlic, rosemary, seaweed	Carrot, comfrey, hemp, olive, sunflower
Hot spots (moist dermatitis, summer sores, wet excema)	Basil, cistus, cedarwood, chamomile (both), helichrysum, lavender, patchouli, rosalina, tea tree, thyme linalol, yarrow	Calendula, olive, sunflower
Infections	Garlic, lavender, lavender white, manuka, rosalina, tea tree, thyme	Calendula, comfrey, neem, olive

Condition	Essential Oils	Carrier Oils
Insect bites	Basil, cistus, chamomile (German), helichrysum, lavender, tansy, yarrow	Hemp, jojoba, olive, sunflower
Lice	Geranium, lemongrass, lavender, rosalina, rosemary, tea tree	Neem, olive
Mange	Bergamot, cistus, chamomile (German), garlic, helichrysum, lavender, lavender white, manuka, rosalina, tea tree, thyme	Neem, calendula, olive
Mosquito	Cistus, geranium, lemongrass, tansy	Neem, calendula
Mud Fever	Garlic, chamomile (German), lavender, lavender white, myrrh, manuka, rosalina, thyme linalol, tea tree, yarrow	Calendula, carrot, neem, jojoba, shea
Proud Flesh	Cistus, chamomile, helichrysum, lavender	Calendula, jojoba
Pyoderma	Chamomile (German), garlic, helichrysum, lavender, tea tree, thyme linalol, yarrow	Calendula, comfrey, neem, olive
Rain Scald	Cistus, chamomile (German), lavender, lavender white, manuka, myrrh, rosalina, thyme linalol, tea tree, yarrow	Calendula, neem, olive
Ringworm	Bergamot, chamomile (German), garlic, helichrysum, lavender, lavender white, manuka, myrrh, rosalina, tea tree	Neem, calendula, jojoba, olive
Sarcoids	Bergamot, carrot seed, cistus, frankincense, lavender, lemon, tea tree	Carrot, calendula, sunflower
Scars	Benzoin, cistus, frankincense, lavender, neroli, yarrow	Calendula, comfrey, hypericum, jojoba
Sebhorrea	Bergamot, cedarwood, geranium	Calendula, jojoba, sunflower
Skin problems	Benzoin (cracked), carrot seed (poor condition), cistus (varied), elemi (older, dry), geranium (flaky, greasy), chamomile (German) (eruptive), lavender, manuka (eruptive), myrrh (damp, oozing), Roman chamomile (stress-related, itchy), yarrow	Calendula, comfrey, hemp, hypericum, jojoba, olive, sesame
Soft lumps	Angelica root, cistus, fennel (sweet), flouve, ginger, grapefruit, hay, lentisk, seaweed	Comfrey, hemp, olive,
Sweet itch	Cistus, cedarwood, geranium, chamomile (both), frankincense, flouve, hay, lavender, tansy, seaweed, yarrow	Calendula, neem, hemp, sunflower, jojoba
Thrush	Eucalyptus, garlic, lavender white, manuka, rosalina, tea tree, thyme	Calendula, sunflower, olive, jojoba
Ticks	Cistus, lemongrass, marjoram, tea tree, patchouli	Neem

Tumours	Bergamot, cistus, fennel (sweet), flouve, frank-incense, hay, juniper berry, lavender, lentisk, lemon, seaweed	Comfrey, hemp, olive, sesame
Ulcers	Frankincense, lentisk, manuka, plai, rosalina, tea tree	Sunflower, calendula, jojoba
Urticaria	Basil, cistus, chamomile (German), helichrysum, flouve, hay, lavender, tansy, yarrow	Calendula, comfrey, hemp, olive
Warts	Bergamot, carrot seed, lavender, lentisk, tea tree	Calendula, jojoba, sunflower

URINARY SYSTEM

Adrenal exhaustion	Angelica root, basil, cedarwood, cypress, frankincense, geranium, lavender white, lemon, seaweed, vetiver, rhododendron	Carrot, olive, sunflower, sesame, hypericum
Bladder infections	Rosalina, bergamot, cajeput, carrot seed, fennel (sweet), patchouli, thyme, yarrow	Olive, sunflower, sesame
Bladder/kidney stones	Basil, fennel, juniper berry, lentisk, lemon	Olive, sunflower, sesame
Inappropriate urination	Bergamot, carrot seed, frankincense, jasmine, lemon, neroli, yarrow, ylang-ylang	Grapeseed, hypericum sunflower, sesame
Incontinence	Benzoin, carrot seed, cedarwood, grapefruit, lemon, patchouli, yarrow	Carrot, hemp, olive, sesame
Kidney Infections	Bergamot, cedarwood, chamomile (German), juniper berry, lemon, plai, rosalina, tea tree, thyme, yarrow	Hemp, hypericum, olive, sesame, sunflower
Kidney deficiency	Angelica root, basil, bergamot, cedarwood, geranium, ginger, lemon, plai, yarrow	Grapeseed, hemp, sesame, sunflower,
FLUTD (feline lower urinary tract disease)	Bergamot, carrot seed, chamomile (German), lemon, thyme linalol, yarrow	Hemp, olive, sunflower, sesame

EARS AND EYES (Do not put essential oils inside ears and eyes, use hydrosols)

Ear infections	Chamomile (German), lavender white, myrrh, yarrow	
Runny eyes	Chamomile, cornflower, rose, sandalwood	
Aural plaque	Myrrh, manuka, lavender, lavender white, rosalina, thyme linalol	Calendula, neem, sunflower
Conjunctivitis	Chamomile (both), cornflower, rose,	
Ear mites	Chamomile (German), lavender, thyme linalol	Calendula, neem
Glaucoma	Carrot seed, hemp	Sunflower
Moon blindness/ recurrent uveitis	Clary sage, hemp, yarrow	Grapeseed, hemp, sunflower

FIRST AID

Abrasions	Cistus, helichrysum, lavender, manuka, rosalina, yarrow	Comfrey, calendula

Abscesses	Garlic, lavender white, manuka, rosalina, tea tree, thyme	Sunflower, olive
Boils	Bergamot, chamomile (German), garlic, helichrysum, lavender white, manuka, lemon, rosalina, seaweed, tea tree, thyme	Calendula, olive, jojoba
Broken Bones	Helichrysum, plai, yarrow	Comfrey
Bruises	Cistus, helichrysum, lavender	Comfrey, sunflower
Burns	Cistus, eucalyptus, helichrysum, lavender	Calendula, olive, hypericum
Cuts	Cistus, helichrysum, lavender, manuka, myrrh, rosalina, tea tree, yarrow	Sunflower, jojoba, calendula
Shock/Hysteria	Lavender, neroli, valerian, ylang-ylang	Undiluted
Sprains & strains	Chamomile (German), helichrysum, lentisk, marjoram, nutmeg, peppermint, plai, rosemary, spearmint, violet leaf, yarrow	Calendula, comfrey
Sunburn	Cistus, lavender, chamomile (Roman), helichrysum, witch hazel hydrosol	Calendula, hypericum, olive
Toxins/poisonous bites	Angelica root, basil, sweet fennel, plai, seaweed, thyme	Calendula, sunflower

BEHAVIOUR/EMOTIONAL
(For behavioural problems use neutral base oils such as sunflower or grapeseed)

Abandonment	Benzoin, carrot seed, lavender white, marjoram, nutmeg
Abuse	Bergamot, carrot seed, helichrysum, rose, seaweed, yarrow
Aggression	Bergamot, hemp, hyssop, jasmine, clary sage, peppermint, thyme
Anger	Bergamot, chamomile (Roman), eucalyptus, helichrysum, rose, yarrow
Anxiety	Benzoin, chamomile (German), clary sage, elemi, frankincense, hemp, jasmine, lavender white, manuka, marjoram, nutmeg, violet leaf, rhododendron
Boredom	Basil, lemon, peppermint, rosemary
Bullying	Bergamot, jasmine, peppermint
Claustrophobia	Cajeput, clary sage, eucalyptus, frankincense, lentisk, rhododendron
Companion (loss)	Cistus, cypress, frankincense, marjoram (sweet), myrrh neroli
Concentration (lack of)	Basil, cedarwood, lemon, nutmeg, peppermint, rosemary

Confidence (lack of)	Cedarwood, ginger, jasmine, rosemary, violet leaf, ylang-ylang
Cribbing	Basil, cajeput, frankincense, lemon, peppermint, vanilla
Crowds (overwhelmed by/restless in)	Juniper berry, lentisk
Depression	Basil, bergamot, cypress, eucalyptus, geranium, ginger, lavender white, lentisk, neroli, nutmeg, orange, rose, thyme
Defensive aggression	Clary sage, frankincense, jasmine, lemon, lentisk peppermint, hyssop, thyme
Disengaged	Basil, benzoin, cistus, juniper berry, flouve, lentisk, myrrh, rosemary
Erratic behaviour	Angelica root, basil, benzoin, bergamot, clary sage, elemi, hemp, vetiver, violet leaf
Fear	Cistus, cedarwood, chamomile (Roman), frankincense, hemp, lemon, jasmine, thyme, valerian, violet leaf, yarrow, ylang-ylang
Flighty	Basil, cedarwood, chamomile (Roman), elemi, hemp, lavender white, lentisk, neroli, nutmeg, patchouli, vetiver, violet leaf
Frustration	Bergamot, chamomile (Roman), clary sage, eucalyptus, lentisk
Hierarchical issues	Jasmine, peppermint, spearmint, ylang-ylang
Hyperactive	Chamomile (Roman), elemi, hemp, lavender, lavaender white, lemon, marjoram, nutmeg, rosemary, vetiver
Impatient	Eucalyptus, chamomile (Roman), clary sage, helichrysum, hemp, jasmine, lemon, lentisk, orange, vanilla
Insecure	Fennel (sweet), geranium, ginger, jasmine, lavender white, marjoram, nutmeg, rose, vetiver, violet leaf
Irritability	Bergamot, chamomile (both), grapefruit, hemp, helichrysum, hyssop, peppermint, orange, tansy
Lethargic	Basil, bergamot, cedarwood, grapefruit, ginger, lemon, lentisk, peppermint, rosemary, thyme
Moodiness	Bergamot, clary sage, geranium, rose, vanilla
Nervous	Angelica root, cistus, basil, cedarwood, chamomile (Roman), clary sage, elemi, frankincense, geranium, jasmine, lavender, orange (sweet), violet leaf, ylang-ylang, valerian, vetiver

New home	Benzoin, cistus, cedarwood, cypress, geranium, lemon, lentisk, violet leaf
Obsessive behaviours	Basil, cajeput, fennel (sweet), hemp, hyssop, vanilla
Pushy	Angelica root, benzoin, hemp, jasmine, nutmeg, vetiver, ylang-ylang
Restless	Clary sage, frankincense, hemp, juniper berry, lavender, lentisk, rose, valerian, vetiver, ylang ylang
Self-harm/mutilation:	Angelica root, basil, cistus, carrot seed, hemp, lemon, neroli, rose, vanilla
Separation anxiety	Angelica root, basil, benzoin, cedarwood, frankincense, hemp, jasmine, lavender, neroli, valerian, ylang-ylang
Shy	Basil, benzoin, cistus, cedarwood, ginger, lavender, thyme
Spraying/Territorial Marking	Bergamot, carrot seed, frankincense, jasmine, neroli, yarrow, ylang-ylang
Suspicious	Cistus, juniper berry, lemon, lentisk, violet leaf
Timid	Cedarwood, cypress, lavender, lemon, thyme, vetiver
Travel phobia	Basil, frankincense, ginger, jasmine, neroli, peppermint
Worry	Benzoin, fennel (sweet), lemon, frankincense, lavender white, marjoram, myrrh, peppermint, spearmint

ESSENTIAL OIL PROFILES (MA3)

Following are profiles of 56 essential oils commonly used with animals. I have limited myself as much as possible to those that I use frequently and are easily available to the dedicated layman. However, there are some oils that are so useful I had to include them even though they are harder to find, such as flouve. The profiles are based on available research and historical usage, my own experience, what the animals have taught me through their selections, and what the plants have transmitted to me when working with them. Use these profiles to gain a deeper understanding of the available aromatics. and develop a feeling of the physical and energetic attributes of this plant, so you can match it to the profile of the animal you are treating. Each profile includes:

The oil's name

The oil profiles are listed alphabetically according to their commonly used names. In brackets below is the Latin name. It is important to know the Latin name because there is sometimes confusion about the common name, or there are two oils with the same name (e.g. chamomile), which are from different plants. Make sure you have the correct oil by checking the Latin name when ordering essential oils.

Element

The element to which the essential oil is most closely aligned. Most oils relate to more than one element, secondary elements are in brackets.

History and Character

The physical description helps you get a picture of where, why and how this plant grows. This helps develop a feeling of the physical and energetic attributes of this plant, so you can match it to the profile of the animal.

Synonyms

Other common names of the plant.

Cultivation/sustainability

It is important to consider how a plant is grown, so you can make considered choices about the ecological impact of the essential oils you use.

Extraction

How the oil is extracted from the plant.

Fragrance

How you can expect the oil to smell.

Principal Constituents

The major chemical constituents that make up the essential oil.

Actions and safety

What the oil does physiologically and any safety precautions that you need to note.

Principal uses

How I have used the oil most frequently with animals, this does not mean it is the only way to use the oil!

Think 'Oil Name' for

Hints to help you match the character of the oil to the character of the 'patient'. These are typical examples of a collection of characteristics that would make you more likely to choose that oil, but do not limit yourself to only that set of circumstances if the oil seems suitable for other reasons.

ANGELICA ROOT

(Angelica Archangelica)

Element: Water (Earth, Fire)

History and Character

Angelica is a large, graceful plant that can grow to a height of 2 metres/6 ft. The whole plant expresses the energetic depth and aspiration that reflects angelica's healing power; its roots go deep into the ground and the large white/green umbrella-like flower is protective. Angelica root oil has long been renowned for its healing powers and was traditionally used to protect against the Plague, for nervous hysteria, as a general tonic, for 'fortifying the spirit', and for female disorders. Angelica opens us to healing, reconnects us to our inner innocence and is said to 'connect us to the angels'. Angelica is innocent and strong at the same time and is very effective where fears and phobias have been triggered by a traumatic incident when very young.

Synonyms

Garden angelica, Holy Spirit Root, Angelica officinalis, and Angel's Herb.

Cultivation/sustainability

Mostly cultivated. No known sustainability issues

Extraction and Characteristics

By steam distillation from roots. The oil is a colourless liquid becoming slightly golden brown as it matures.

Fragrance

Sweet, sharp, pungent, with earthy undertones.

Principal Constituents

Terpenes: α-pinene, 3-carene, limonene, β-myrcene, α-phellandrene. A-caryophyllene, camphene, β-phellandrene, copaene, β-pinene, γ-terpinene
Esters: bornyl acetate
Coumarins: bergapten

Actions

Antifungal, antispasmodic, antitoxic, antibacterial, carminative, digestive, diuretic, expectorant, febrifuge, general tonic, neurotonic.

Safety

Non-toxic, non-irritant. Angelica root oil can be photo-toxic when applied to skin undiluted; avoid exposure to sun for 12 hours after topical application. Avoid use with diabetes.

Principal Uses

Physical
   » Animals who have shut down due to chronic pain or stress
   » Arthritis
   » Chronic bronchial disorders
   » Circulatory problems
   » Cushing's syndrome and other metabolic disorders
   » Immune stimulant, especially for those run down by a long illness
   » Liver dysfunction
   » Loss of appetite, including anorexia
   » Lymphatic problems
   » Stress-related digestive disorders

Behavioural
   » Chronic anxiety
   » Fears born out of early childhood trauma
   » Strengthens the nerves, especially where there is hysteria brought on by nervous exhaustion

Think 'Angelica' for:

Uncontrollable fears, especially after a traumatic incident in early life
Old animals who are emotionally hardened or have chronic pain
If an animal shows no interest in any of the oils offered to it.

BASIL, SWEET

(Ocimum Basilicum)

Element: Earth (Fire)

History and Character:

The basil plant is familiar to most of us as a common kitchen herb. This variety, Ocimum Basilicum, has glossy green leaves with a sharp, pungent aroma, and a sharp spike of purple flowers. The herb's name is said to derive from the Greek for King, so it is sometimes known as the royal herb and is said to give courage. In India they more commonly use Holy Basil or Tulsi (Basilicum sanctum), which is considered sacred and is a Hindu symbol of love, eternal life, purification and protection with a wide range of medicinal uses. However essential oil from Ocimum sanctum is high in eugenol and less safe to use than common basil. Ocimum basilicum grows wild all over the sunny hillsides of the Mediterranean where it is used traditionally for respiratory problems, digestive problems, and to protect against malaria and other feverish epidemics. It is also used as an antidote to poisonous snake and insect bites. Although this oil is vibrant and energetically dynamic it is also cooling, but should be used in small amounts. It cools hotheads, focussing the mind and clearing emotional reactivity.

Synonyms

Joy of the Mountain, Boy Joy, True sweet basil.

Cultivation/sustainability

Cultivated

Extraction and Characteristics

Steam distillation of leaves and flowering tops. A light, clear to yellow oil.

Fragrance

Fresh sweet, pungent, green, with balsamic undertones.

Principal Constituents

(Quantities vary considerably, depending on chemotype.)

Terpenes: pinene, limonene, camphene

Alcohols: linalol

Phenolic ethers: methyl chavicol

Actions

Adrenal cortex stimulant, analgesic, antibacterial, antidepressant, antiseptic, antiviral, carminative, cephalic, expectorant, febrifuge, galactagogue, neurotonic, nervous system regulator, restorative, tonic, uterine decongestant.

Safety

Relatively non-toxic, non-irritant, possible sensitisation in some individuals. Use in high dilutions. There is also 'exotic' basil which is high in methyl chavicol and considered unsafe to use in aromatherapy.

Principal Uses

Physical:
  » Congested coughs and colds especially if fever is present
  » Insect bites
  » Muscle cramps
  » Sluggish circulation
  » Tired overworked muscles
  » Viral infections

Behavioural:
  » Flighty, distracted animals
  » Head shaking
  » Lack of concentration
  » Those that fall apart under pressure
  » Travel phobia

Think 'Basil' for:

Nervous animals who lack concentration or 'play the fool' but can become hysterical if pushed, especially if they have digestive or muscle problems.
Reactions to toxins or poisonous bites.

BENZOIN RESINOID

(Benzoin Styrax)

Element: Earth

History and Character

It is a common member of the forests of South East Asia, where it grows to about 12-30 (40-100 feet) meters in height. Styrax benzoin can live 70-100 years and thrives in mountainous areas and cold temperatures with high rainfall. The resin naturally seeps out of the tree's trunk when it is cut, to protect it from invasive bacteria. This resin is collected and dried for use as incense and for medicinal purposes. One of benzoin's traditional uses was in Friar's balsam, an inhalant for coughs and colds. Ballet dancers used it for cracked feet. It was said to 'drive out evil spirits', which is an old fashioned way of describing any remedy that had a powerful psychological effect. Benzoin has a calming and strengthening affect on the psyche and is a very comforting oil. One of the principal qualities of this oil is stabilising, bringing the user into their belly and out of their intellect, relaxing the mind and strengthening the being. One of its key functions is to strengthen physically and psychologically and is good for those who feel they carry too heavy a load, or tend to take on the worries and anxieties of others.

Benzoin, unblocks the bucker

One of the first times I used benzoin was with a horse who had injured himself some years before and seemed unable to reconnect with the injured area, where the scar ran along his side. Anything that caused him to think about this area such as being groomed, the rider's leg touching it, or turning to the right, could cause an angry reaction and he regularly bucked his rider off. It was so extreme that when I first stood and looked at the scar, from about 2 ft away, the horse became fidgety and tried to bite his owner. I offered the horse benzoin, which he breathed deeply, going into a slight trance. Then, with a few drops of diluted benzoin on my hands, I brushed the scar very lightly, two or three times, not even touching the skin. The horse breathed out loudly turned to look at me and touched the scar with his nose. From then on he was happy to be handled from the right, as if there had never been a problem.

Synonyms
Gum Benzoin, Gum Benjamin.

Cultivation/sustainability
Many trees are cultivated for resin extraction, but in the wild they are listed as vulnerable.

Extraction and Characteristics
Benzoin is not strictly speaking an essential oil but a resin. It is collected directly from the tree, but to make it useable commercially it is dissolved in ethyl alcohol. You can also use the resin directly if you heat it until it melts.

Fragrance
Warm, sweet, vanilla with a woody resinous edge.

Principal Constituents
Esters: coniferyl cinnamate, coniferyl benzoate, benzyl cinnamate
Acids: benzoic acid, cinnaminic acid, plus other acids
Aldehydes: benzaldehyde, vanillin

Actions
Anti-inflammatory, antioxidant, antiseptic, astringent, carminative, diuretic, expectorant, sedative, styptic, vulnerary.

Safety
Non-toxic, non-irritant, possible sensitisation in some individuals.

Principal Uses

Physical:

- » Any invasion of cold or damp
- » Arthritis
- » Coughs and colds, especially if mucous lingers
- » Dry, cracked skin or feet
- » Nervous stomach
- » Weak back, or lack of backbone

Behavioural:

- » Over thinking and worry, over-concern for others
- » Trauma associated with old scars

Think 'Benzoin' for:

Animals who become anxious, withdrawn or distracted when separated from intimates, especially if they suffer from dry skin or 'lack backbone', or are prone to self injury.

Emotional or physical reactivity due to physical or emotional scars.

BERGAMOT

(Citrus Bergamia)

Element: Wood (Water)

History and Character

Named for the city of Bergamo in Italy this small tree (3.5 metres/12' high) resembles a miniature orange. Traditionally it was used in Italy for fever and worms, also to stop the spread of infection in hospitals as it is said to kill airborne bacteria. One of the main qualities of bergamot is its balancing affect. This is particularly useful where things are out of control, as in growths, tumours and, on an emotional level, moods that swing between extremes. Bergamot's sharp, sweet smell is uplifting and clean, cutting through stagnant energies to release pent up emotion. It has a profound antidepressant effect, especially for those individuals who turn anger and frustration in on themselves, which can manifest in animals as self-mutilation or obsessive compulsive behaviour.

Synonyms

Citrus aurantium subsp. Bergamia. There is a herb known as bergamot (or bee balm) that is no relation.

Cultivation/sustainability

Cultivated. Use organic cultivation

Extraction and Characteristics

Cold-pressed from the skin of the fruit. The oil is a clear green colour.

Fragrance
A fresh, citrus aroma with a slightly green edge.

Principal Constituents
Esters: linalyl acetate, geranyl acetate
Alcohols: linalol, geraniol
Terpenes: limonene, ß-pinene, γ-terpinene, ρ-cymene, δ-3-carene
Furocoumarin: bergapten

Actions
Antibacterial, antiseptic, antispasmodic, antiviral, calmative, cicatrizant, febrifuge, parasiticide, sedative, stomachic, tonic, vermifuge.

Safety
Whole bergamot oil is photo–toxic so should not be applied to exposed skin up to 12 hours before exposure to ultra violet. Otherwise it is non-toxic and relatively non-irritant. It is possible to buy bergapten–free bergamot, but I never use it, because animals consistently choose the whole oil over the altered one.

Principal Uses

Physical:
  » Endocrine balance
  » Genito-urinary tract infections
  » Post parturition
  » Ringworm
  » Tumours, warts, sarcoids, growths of all kinds
  » Viral infection

Behavioural:
  » Depression
  » Frustrated irritability
  » Snappiness

Think 'Bergamot' for:
Sarcoids, growths and tumours, especially if the animal is snappy, intolerant or withdrawn. Changeable, moody individuals with unpredictable temperament.

CAJEPUT

(Melaleuca Cajeputi Powell)

Element: Metal

History and Character

Cajeput is a tall evergreen tree with thick pointed leaves and white flowers native to Indonesia, Malaysia, South-east Asia and tropical Australia. Traditionally it has been used for joint pain, earache, respiratory problems and for repelling head lice and fleas. Cajeput is also known as white tea tree and is from the same family as tea tree and rosalina; it shares the energetic sharpness and disinfectant properties of these oils. As with many of the Metal oils, cajeput focuses and cleanses energetic space. It can be useful in cutting through obsessive behaviours by sharpening the mind and freeing it from a sense of entrapment.

Synonyms

Cajuput, White Tea Tree, White Wood, Swamp Tea Tree, Punk Tree, Paperbark Tree.

Cultivation/sustainability

Mostly cultivated. Wild population healthy

Extraction and Characteristics

Steam distilled from the fresh leaves and twigs. The oil is a pale yellowy-green liquid.

Fragrance

Camphoraceous, 'medicinal', with a slightly fruity edge.

Principal Constituents

Oxides: 1,8-cineole
Terpenes: β-pinene, limonene, β-caryophyllene, α-pinene
Alcohols: α-terpineol

Actions

Antirheumatic, antiseptic, antispasmodic, expectorant, febrifuge, insecticide, pulmonary disinfectant, tonic and stimulant.

Safety

Non-toxic, non-sensitising but can irritate skin in high concentrations. For topical application dilute well. Avoid contact with mucous membranes.

Aggie's aggravated ears

By Deb Heubert, Animal Holistic Health Practitioner, Animal PsychAromaticist, Wisconsin USA

Aggie, a 6-year-old spayed Chocolate Lab with a chronic ear infection which despite antibiotic treatment made her shake her head violently and scratch her eyes till they bled.

In Chinese terms, Aggie was exhibiting excess Heat and Damp in her body, indicated by the on-going fungal infection. This was partly an outcome of a diet based on cereals and dry food. She was also experiencing mental stress, in part triggered by the introduction of a new puppy into the household and her feeling the need to assume an alpha role.

Aggie needed cooling, drying oils that would help restore balance. Oils selected were bergamot, antibacterial, skin balancing and a strong antidepressant, for those that turn anger and frustration inward, it also harmonizes Liver Qi, aiding digestion; lavender, soothes skin, regulates and cools an overheated liver; helichrysum, soothes itching skin and releases blocked energy, especially anger that has turned to depression.

Aggie's food was changed to fresh meat (cooked or raw), brown rice and a variety of vegetables, plus a good vitamin/herbal supplement along with probiotics and enzymes. Aggie's owners were given several easy behavioural modifications, to relieve her anxiety. Her ears were wiped with calendula oil and lavender essential oil (1 drop to 5 ml). These oils are soothing, antibacterial, anti-fungal and healing.

Aggie showed interest in helichrysum for three months, by then the redness around her nose and eyes was gone and hair had regrown around her muzzle. The black oozing matter from her ears had disappeared and she had stopped scratching them. She was obviously happier and stopped turning away when someone wanted to pet her..

Principal Uses

Physical:
- » Circulatory problems and arthritis
- » Coughs and viral infections of the lungs
- » General immune tonic

Behavioural:
- » Obsessive compulsive behaviours

Think "Cajeput" for:

Animals exhibiting obsessive behaviours, such as dogs tail chasing or horses cribbing, especially if they have breathing problems or a tendency to lung infections.

CARROT SEED

(Daucus Carota)

Element: Earth (Wood, Water)

History and Character

Wild carrot has a graceful, white flower growing from a succulent root, similar to the yellow carrot we know so well but smaller and paler. The finest carrot seed essential oil is wild-harvested in France, where the plant can be found in the fields and hedgerows of rural areas. The oil is well accepted by all types of animal and is highly nourishing, physically and emotionally. Carrot seed regenerates liver cells, helps repair damaged skin, rebuilds poor quality hooves and nails, and encourages the production of healthy tissue in smooth muscles. I often use it where an animal has, or has had, a high worm load, as it is a vermifuge and helps repair damage to the stomach lining. Because of its high levels of nutrients, this is the oil to use if there is any history of physical or emotional neglect, abandonment or starvation. Because of its connection to nourishment, it is a good oil for loss of appetite and the loss of appetite for life. Like a true earth mother it responds to our needs and helps rebuild the system from the inside out.

Synonyms

Wild Carrot, Queen Anne's lace, Birds Nest.

Cultivation/sustainability

Most essential oil comes from cultivated plants. Wild population healthy

Extraction and Characteristics

Steam distilled from the dried seeds.

Fragrance

Damp earth, sweet, musty, warm.

Principal Constituents

Terpenes: α-pinene, sabinene
Esters: geranyl acetate
Alcohols: carotol, daucol, geraniol, terpinen-4-ol

Actions

Anthelmintic, antiseptic, carminative, detoxicant, diuretic, emmenagogue, hepatic, regenerative, smooth muscle relaxant, stimulant, tonic, vasodilator.

Safety

Generally non-toxic, non-sensitising. Can be harsh on skin, dilute well.

Principal Uses

Physical:

- » Anorexia
- » Flatulence
- » Heart murmurs
- » Liver damage
- » Loss of appetite
- » Malnutrition (past or present)
- » Poor skin and hooves
- » Slow-healing wounds
- » Ulcers
- » Worms

Behavioural:

- » Emotional neglect or abandonment
- » Loss of will to live

Think 'Carrot Seed' for:

Any time there is or has been abandonment or neglect, emotional or physical.

An inability to give or receive nurture, especially if the animal is underweight or heals slowly or has a poor quality coat or hooves/nails.

Feeling abandoned calls for carrot seed

I was asked to treat a retired school horse, who was feeling depressed. Once he had been the star of the school, but was now getting on in years and his owner had better horses for the job. So he had been retired out to pasture with another horse. But despite the good grass, Pancho was losing weight and spent much of his time alone. In fact, Pancho viewed his honourable retirement as abandonment and was feeling depressed. The oils chosen for him were neroli, for its uplifting effect, and carrot seed for his feeling of abandonment and to help him put on weight. He showed interest in the neroli for 3 days, inhaling it, and the carrot seed for a week, licking and sniffing. Within two days he was much brighter and socialising more. At the end of a week his coat looked better, he was starting to gain weight, and his owner had realised he still had much to offer her students with his patience and wisdom, even if he could not master advanced lateral work, so she put him back into light work.

CEDARWOOD ATLAS

(Cedrus Atlantica)

Element: Water (Metal)

History and Character

This magnificent tree is graceful and powerful with an awesome presence. It is native to the Atlas Mountains of Morocco and thought to be related to the Cedar of Lebanon. It is also closely related to the Himalayan cedar (Cedrus deodara), which produces an essential oil that can be used interchangeably with the Atlas cedar. Cedarwood has a long tradition of religious use in various cultures as an incense and for building temples. the Egyptians used it for embalming and cosmetics. The cedarwood tree grows in high mountains, where the air is clean and fresh, the tree has deep spreading roots and a tall straight trunk, the branches are flexible, moving in the wind but anchored to the central trunk. Cedarwood oil grounds and centres you in your being, encouraging you to take a deep breath so you have the strength to face up to every situation. It helps those who feel alienated, or fear they don't have the strength to 'hold it together', or feel overwhelmed by circumstances they have no control over. Cedarwood gives inner calm in times of instability and is one of the oils to try if you are moving house or your animal's environment is disturbed in any way.

Synonyms

Atlantic Cedar, Atlas Cedar, African Cedar, Moroccan Cedarwood.

Cultivation/sustainability

Prefer to purchase from cultivated sources

Extraction and Characteristics

Steam distillation from wood, stumps and sawdust. It is a yellow, amber viscous oil.

Fragrance

A warm, woody, slightly camphoraceous odour.

Principal Constituents

Terpenes: himachalenes cadinene gurjenene
Ketones: α-eglantine
Numerous other trace compounds

Actions

Anticatarrhal, antiparasitic, antirheumatic, anti-seborrhoea, cicatrisant, diuretic, expectorant, general tonic, lymphatic decongestant.

Safety

Non-toxic and non-irritant in prescribed doses.

Principal Uses

Physical:
- » Asthma
- » Catarrh
- » Hair loss
- » Insect repellent
- » Oedema
- » Weak kidneys or back
- » Wheezing

Behavioural:
- » Fear, timidity
- » Lack of willpower
- » New home or moving house

Think 'Cedarwood' for:

Those who are unsettled by their surroundings or have moved home.

Timid fearful animals, especially if there is a history of back ache, kidney problems or hair loss.

CHAMOMILE, GERMAN

(Matricaria Recutita)

Element: Wood (Earth)

History and Character

German chamomile grows up to 60 cm (2') tall, with a branching stem that bears sprays of small white flowers with a pale yellow centre. It is similar in action to Roman chamomile, but more powerfully anti-inflammatory and anti-allergenic,. It is one of the most anti-inflammatory essential oils. It also soothes irritated skin. Emotionally, German chamomile soothes anxiety and is useful for those who tend to express their emotions through their body, getting ill rather than getting upset. German chamomile is especially good for animals who are stoic and don't show their feelings easily. One of this oil's most useful actions is its ability to clear Damp Heat and unblock the flow of energy in the body, so there is often a squishy or stodgy feel or look to animals who need German chamomile. The deep blue colour of this oil is due to the chamazulene, which is an anti-inflammatory agent and an outcome of the distillation process.

Synonyms

Blue Chamomile, Hungarian Chamomile, Sweet False Chamomile.

Cultivation/sustainability

Cultivated. Healthy wild population

German chamomile for overheating

Mel, a 15-year–old quarter horse/paint mare, had suffered from itchy skin since she was three years old. Every summer she rubbed off all her mane and tail and tore her skin on her chest. She lived in an electrified pen and stable to stop her rubbing, which increased her stress levels. It also meant she could never be turned out with the herd. Mel was also constantly in heat, spraying the backs of her legs with the acidic excretions mare's urinate when in season. She was very attached to her stable mate, a young gelding, and became highly anxious when he was taken away from her, even if he was still in view. She was always slightly grumpy and depressed.

Mel's main imbalance was the Liver meridian. She was offered German chamomile, geranium and rose otto, each diluted in calendula macerated oil. I also made a lotion from pink clay, rose hydrolat, geranium and chamomile essential oils, and neem oil. The lotion was applied to her body where she indicated (mostly on her head, chest and tail) for relief from the itching, and protection from flies. Within a few days of starting the oils, Mel's hormonal cycle normalised and her itching decreased. She took these first oils for about a month, by the end of which she was only itching on days of extremely hot weather. A year later, some dietary changes and the oils, and Mel is itch free, all year.

Extraction and Characteristics
Steam distilled from the dried flower heads. The oil is a deep blue.

Fragrance
Sweet, herbaceous and bitter.

Principal Constituents
Alcohols: α-bisabolol, α-bisabolol oxide A,
α-bisabolol oxide B, bisabolone oxide A
Terpenes: chamazulene, trans-α-farnesene, trans-β-farnesene, δ-cadinene

Actions
Analgesic, anti-allergenic, antifungal, anti-inflammatory, antispasmodic, bactericidal, digestive, emmenagogue, hepatic, nerve sedative, stimulates leucocyte production, vulnerary.

Safety
Generally held to be non-toxic and non-irritant. Can cause contact dermatitis in some individuals.

Principal Uses

Physical:
- » Allergies effecting skin or lungs
- » Arthritis
- » Eruptive skin conditions
- » First heat or season
- » Fungal infection
- » Insect bites
- » Soft tissue swellings
- » Spasmodic colic
- » Ulcers

Behavioural:
- » Anxiety
- » Impatience
- » Irritability

Think "German Chamomile" for:

Sweet itch and other allergic skin reactions especially if the animal is worn down and irritable. Fungal infections and Stomach Heat (ulcers).

CHAMOMILE, ROMAN

(Anthemis Nobilis, Chamamaelum Nobile)

Element: Wood

History and Character

Roman Chamomile is a small, half-spreading herb with feathery leaves and daisy like flowers; a sweet and gentle plant, delicate yet sturdy. Native to southern and western Europe, it is widely cultivated throughout Europe and the USA. This pale blue oil, is similar to its cousin German chamomile, but less anti-inflammatory and more suited to those who are likely to make a fuss about every little thing, rather than bear it stoically. Roman chamomile is ideal for those who are constitutionally nervous, 'jumping out of their skins' and over-reactive, especially if they suffer from diarrhoea when anxious. The oil calms the nerves, stomach and skin, and helps them live more comfortably in their skins, physically and emotionally. For me it is "the child's oil" as it is gentle, soothing and works well for 'growing up' problems, such as teething, colic and restlessness. It also helps animals who are fearful or nervous with children and soothes immature tantrums and outbursts of emotion, however old you are.

Synonyms

English Chamomile, Garden Chamomile, True Chamomile, Sweet Chamomile.

Cultivation/sustainability

Cultivated. Healthy wild population

Extraction and Characteristics

Steam distillation of the flower heads. A pale, blue, mobile liquid, turning yellow with age.

Roman Chamomile for serenity

Courtesy of Wendy Wolfe, Animal Wellness Educator

Serena was a young, blonde, Chinese Crested dog that had been rescued from a puppy mill raid. Her person brought her to me because, in spite of her efforts, she could not get Serena to relax. Serena was frightened of everything and everyone and visibly shook most of the time. As she sat in my office she trembled terribly. I offered her Chamomile (Roman), 1 drop diluted in 5 ml of Safflower oil. She inhaled it deeply and looked off into space. She inhaled again and within two minutes the trembling stopped. She relaxed, lay her head down on the floor and took a much needed rest. Her person continued to offer her the Roman Chamomile twice a day for about two weeks. Once Serena was calm and energetically in her body, she came to excel in agility and became a happy pack member. Serena's vet, said he had never witnessed such a change in a dog.

Fragrance
Fruity, herbaceous, apple-like, with a bitter note.

Principal Constituents
Esters: tiglates, angelates
Ketones: pinocarvone
Terpenes: α-pinene, β-pinene, chamazulene

Actions
Analgesic, anti-inflammatory, anti-neuralgic, antiparasitic, antiseptic, antispasmodic, carminative, digestive, sedative, tonic, vulnerary.

Safety
Generally non-toxic and non-irritant; can cause dermatitis in some individuals.

Principal Uses:

Physical:
  » Diarrhoea
  » Excema
  » Inflamed, itchy skin
  » Nervous digestive problems
  » Stress related skin problems
  » Sweet itch

Behavioural:
  » Constitutional nervousness
  » Fear, nervousness or intolerance of children
  » Nervous aggression
  » Restlessness

Think "Roman Chamomile" for:

Nervous flighty animals, especially if they suffer from itchy, irritable skin, or stress related stomach upset.

Any issues that involves children, and frustration or angry outbursts.

CHASTETREE

(Vitex agnus castus)

Element: Earth (Fire)

History and Character

Vitex agnus castus, commonly called chastetree or monks pepper, belongs to the Verbenaceae family. Originating from the Mediterranean basin, it is a branching deciduous shrub, growing up to 3 metres high. The berries are harvested in autumn, as the leaves drop. The plant prefers low altitudes and is often found and is often found along sandy lake shores and riverbeds, and by the sea.

Chastetree has a long historical use. In Greek mythology, Hera, wife of Zeus and the protectoress of matrimony, was said to be born under a chastetree, hence the name. Traditionally the berries were used to reduce sexual desire in celibate monks. Hippocrates (400 BC) recommends the drug for injuries, inflammations and enlargements of the spleen. According to Pliny the Elder (AD. 23-79) V. "it checks violent sexual desire in men, takes away the more severe type of headache, purges the uterus and the bowels. Because of their hot nature, the seeds are taken to dispel flatulence, promote urine, regulate diarrhea and greatly benefit epilepsy and spleen disease."

Nowadays extracts of the berry or leaf are prescribed for a range of hormonal problems in women, and also for prostate enlargement in men. The berries are used in Egypt as a mild sedative, to calm nervous hysteria. Scientific research says vitex's mechanism of action is through its regulatory effect on the endocrine system, particularly the pituitary gland, which in turn generates proper equilibrium of estrogen and progesterone in the body. It also binds to opiate receptors, so has some pain calming activity. Vitex has been used successfully in the management of metabolic syndrome in horses and is one of the most effective hormone balancers, especially for mature females.

Energetically, the the oil is very Yin supportive, grounding and earthy and can be used for Deficient Yin, or Excess Yang. It helps you persevere and find the inner strength to support yourself and others in difficult tasks. It also encourages patience and receptivity. Animals often prefer the hydrosol to the essential oil.

Synonyms
Vitex, chaste tree, chasteberry, Abraham's balm, lilac chastetree, or monk's pepper

Cultivation/sustainability
Wildly cultivated. Healthy wild population

Extraction
Steam distilled from berries or leaves (aerial parts). Berries are more powerful, but less tolerated. A pale yellow to colourless liquid

Fragrance
Musty, river bottom, to floral sweet

Principal Constituents
Terpenes:, 1,8 cineole, α-pinene, β-pinene, Farnesene, trans-Caryolphyllene, α-Copaene, Bicyclogermacrene.
Alcohols and esters α-Terpinyl acetate, Terpinen-4-ol

Actions
Analgesic, anti-inflammatory, anti-spasmodic, hepatic stimulant, hormone regulator, nervine

Safety
Do not use in pregnancy. Dilute well

Principal uses
Physical
- » Metabolic issues
- » Endocrine imbalance (thyroid, pituitary)
- » Enlarged prostate
- » Infertility
- » Irregular seasons (too much/too little)
- » Itching
- » Flatulence

Behavioural
- » Unpredictable
- » Moody mares
- » Sluggish and despairing
- » Nervous and intolerant
- » Bad-tempered

Think 'Chastetree ' for
Any metabolic imbalance, especially if the animal is intolerant or quick-tempered.

CISTUS (CISTUS LADANIFERUS)

Element: Metal

History and Character:

Cistus ladanifer is a species of flowering plant in the family Cistaceae. It is native to the western Mediterranean region, being particularly prolific in Portugal and Spain, where it has taken over much of what was once farmland and grasslands in the mountain regions. The leaves are evergreen and lanceolate, dark green above and paler underneath. The flowers have 5 papery white petals, usually with a red to maroon spot at the base, surrounding the yellow stamens and pistils. The whole plant is covered with sticky, fragrant resin. The plant is known as a pioneer species, moving into repair land that has been degraded, especially if it is cracked and dry.

It is a sturdy shrub, flourishing in harsh environments, yet bears a profusion of delicate white flowers that bloom and fade quickly, thus it symbolises both softness, transience and endurance. The shrub shelters seedlings of other species in its shade, and has a symbiotic relationship with a special root fungi that helps it flourish in arid areas by increasing its ability to take up water. It is self-fertile.

Cistus is one of the plants known as Rose of Sharon, and is possibly the burning bush in the biblical story of Moses. Historically, in Greek and Turkish Folk Medecine, Cistus were used for a great variety of ointments,potions and infusions for everything from the plague, scurvy and hair loss to rheumatism and asthma, although it is unclear which variety this was.

Traditionally, the gum was collected by goat-herders, as the goat's hair became loaded with the resin as they foraged between the shrubs. The coat was sheared and then boiled to retrieve the oleo-resin, which was turned into an absolute, called labdanum, for the fragrancing industry. Supposedly shepherds noticed that working with the resin helped small cuts on their hands heal more quickly. The essential oil is steam distilled from the twigs and leaves and is one of the best skin healing agents, reducing scarring.

Cistus helps those who have shut themselves off and become emotionally cold, due to past trauma or feeling unwanted. The cistus type can seem self-reliant and finds it hard to trust other, but at the same time they struggle to contain their emotions, and over-respond to stimuli. I have found it clears deeply held generational trauma, allowing animals to move past behaviours they are carrying from birth.

Synonyms:

Rock rose, Esteva, gum rockrose, laudanum, labdanum, gum cistus, brown-eyed rockrose.

Cultivation/sustainability

Wildcrafted. Healthy wild population, considered a weed.

Extraction and Characteristics:
Steam distillation of the leaves and flowers. Golden/yellow.

Fragrance:
Balsamic, sweet, woody, flowery
Principal Constituents: a-pinene, camphene, hexen-1-ol, trimetylcyclohexanone, bornyl acetat

Actions:
Antiseptic, anti-infectious, anti-microbial, antiviral, bactericidal, anti-inflammatory, antitussive, astringent, calming, cicatrisant, mucolytic, styptic, tonic for the nervous system, vulnerary

Safety:
No known cautions

Principal uses:
Physical:
» Adrenal exhaustion
» Arthritis
» Catarrhal coughs
» Immune modulated diseases
» Nervous diarrhoea
» Nervous exhaustion,
» Old scars
» Possibly, Metabolic Syndrome
» Restlessness
» Sarcoids
» Sores
» Stiff/cold limbs
» Sweet itch, mud fever
» Ulcers
» Wheezing,
» Wounds

Behavioural:
» After any traumatic incident to clear the nervous system
» emotional detachment
» hysteria
» Lack of self expression
» Nervousness
» Over-submissive

Think "Cistus" for:
Older animals with chronic skin problems, especially if they are emotionally cold or detached, or suffer from the cold,
Animals who over-respond emotionally, especially if they have respiratory problems, or a history of past abuse or abandonment,
Wounds

CLARY SAGE

(Salvia Sclarea)

Element: Metal

History and Character

Clary sage is a sturdy perennial herb with hairy, pale-green, purple-tinged leaves and insignificant blue flowers. It is native to southern Europe but cultivated worldwide wherever the soil is well-drained. In the Middle Ages it was known as Cleareye, which refers both to its ability to cleanse the eyes (the herb, not the essential oil) and its reputation for inducing visions. It is closely related to garden sage (Salvia officinalis), but much safer to use as it has lower levels of ketones. Clary sage is deeply relaxing for muscles and mind; it is euphoric, lifting you above daily cares but at the same time grounding, earthy and inspiring. It is said to have a progesterone like effect and can be used to regulate hormonal cycles and relieve the discomfort of heats or season. It also helps to release energy in the lower chakras, encouraging sexual activity. Last but not least, clary sage releases constriction in the lungs, deepening breathing and relieving fearful tension.

Synonyms:

Clary Wort, Muscatel Sage, Clear Eye, Eye Bright, See Bright. Not to be confused with Salvia officinalis, S. Lavendulaefolia, or the herb Eyebright, which is Euphrasia.

Cultivation/sustainability

Cultivated

Extraction and Characteristics

Steam distillation of the flowering tops and leaves.

Fragrance

Warm, musky, sweet, green and camphoraceous.

Principal Constituents

Esters: linalyl acetate, geranyl acetate, neryl acetate
Alcohols: linalol, sclareol, geraniol, α-terpineol
Terpenes: germacrene D, β-caryophyllene, myrcene, trans-ocimene

Actions

Antifungal, antiseptic, antispasmodic, antisudorific, detoxicant, decongestant, hormone balancer (progesterone-like), neurotonic, phlebotonic, regenerative.

Safety
Non–toxic, non-irritant, non-sensitising. Do not use in pregnancy.

Principal Uses

Physical:
- » Alopecia
- » Asthma
- » Circulatory problems
- » Claustrophobia
- » Hormonal problems
- » Tight or strained muscles

Behavioural:
- » Anxiety
- » Changeable moods
- » Claustrophobia
- » Depression
- » Fear

Think 'Clary Sage' for:
Restless, moody animals, especially if there is any constriction of lungs or muscles, or claustrophobia.

Bad-tempered females, especially if they are defensive of their personal space, or become moody or uncomfortable around their hormonal cycle.

CYPRESS

(Cupressus Sempervirens)

Element: Metal (Water)

History and Character
The evergreen cypress tree is picturesque and graceful with its slender, conical shape and dark-green needles. Its needle-sharp finger pointing darkly at the sky is a defining feature of the Mediterranean landscape. Native to the eastern Mediterranean, it grows wild throughout southern Europe and North Africa. It has been associated with cleansing and transformation (death and renewal) by the Greeks, who dedicated it to Pluto lord of the underworld, and planted it in graveyards as a symbol of continuity. The oil helps us to deal with all change of an inner or outer nature by "strengthening the 'Metal' function of letting in and letting go, and to unearth the fears that block change" (G.Mojay). Cypress controls excessive flow of fluids such as perspiration and tears; it also moves blocked water, such as in oedema or repressed grief. Cypress says: "Have a good cry, then mop up your tears and move on!"

Synonyms
Italian Cypress, Mediterranean Cypress.

Cultivation/sustainability
No sustainability issues

Cypress for life after death

I was giving a talk at a dog-groomers convention once, and in the front row was a small dog who had come to help demonstrate how to use oils. All we could see of this dog was his nose as he hid under a chair. This dog's person had recently died. He had been adopted by her friend straightaway, but he had lost confidence in himself, was very timid and scared of his surroundings. This was new or exaggerated behaviour.

It is difficult to demonstrate animal self selection when your subject won't come out from under the chair. However, I held the open bottle of Cypress in my hand at an unobtrusive distance. Slowly the dog's head crept forward until we could see his nostrils twitching as he inhaled the oil. When the head withdrew, I closed the bottle and continued talking, until I was seriously upstaged by the little dog walking along the front row and greeting everybody. A heart-warming moment indeed.

Extraction and Characteristics
Steam distillation from the needles and twigs. The oil is a pale yellow colour.

Fragrance
Fresh, sweet, coniferous, with a deeper resinous bottom note.

Principal Constituents
Terpenes: α-pinene, δ-3-carene, terpinolene, limonene, δ-cadinene, sabinene, β-pinene, ρ-cymene
Alcohols: borneol, cedrol, α-terpineol
Esters: α-terpenyl acetate

Actions
Antibacterial, antiseptic, antispasmodic, antisudorific, antitussive, astringent, calmative, deodorant, diuretic, hormone-like (ovarian problems), neurotonic, phlebotonic.

Safety
Generally held to be non-toxic, non-irritant and non-sensitising.

Principal Uses

Physical:

» Adrenal regulator
» Asthma
» Back ache
» Excessive or deficient perspiration
» Hormone problems, especially irregular cycles
» Insect repellent
» Muscular cramp
» Oedema, sluggish circulation

Behavioural:

» Animals that have shut down due to moving too much
» Any personal loss that has destabilised emotions
» Easily overwhelmed
» Grief
» Stiff and untrusting
» Timid

Think 'Cypress' for:

Animals who want to move on but are stuck in old behaviour patterns.

Animals whose emotions have been destabilised by death or some other traumatic break in the pattern of life, especially if it manifests as an extreme of behaviour, excessive or inappropriate urination or hormonal problems.

ELEMI

(Canarium Luzonicum)

Element: Metal

History and Character:

Elemi is a tall tropical tree native to the Philippines and the Moluccas, known by the locals as Pili. The bark exudes a green, resinous gum that is made mainly of resin and essential oil, and has been traditionally used in lacquers and fragrances. The name elemi is said to be derived from the Arabic for 'As above, so below' (P.Davies), and energetically this is a balancing oil bringing body, mind and soul into alignment. Like many resinous oils, elemi heals skin, especially older or cracked, dry skin. It is also a bronchial disinfectant. Physically, elemi has similar actions to frankincense, and has often been thought of as poor man's frankincense, but elemi's balancing quality is unique and I find it lighter and more focussed than frankincense.

Synonyms

Manila, Elemi Gum, C. Commune.

Cultivation/sustainability

Wildcrafted. Listed as vulnerable because of destruction of habitat.

Extraction and Characteristics
Steam distillation from the gum. The oil is a pale yellow to brownish liquid.

Fragrance
A light, balsamic, lemony top note and a warm, spicy bottom note.

Principal Constituents
Terpenes: phellandrene, dipentene, limonene, elemicine
Alcohols: elemol, terpineol

Actions
Antiseptic, cicatrisant, expectorant, fortifying, regulatory, stimulant, stomachic, tonic.

Safety
Generally held to be non-toxic, non-irritant and non-sensitising.

Principal Uses

Physical:
- » Asthma
- » Cracked skin
- » Dry coughs with no apparent cause
- » Dry skin
- » Immune compromised
- » Run down

Behavioural:
- » Easily distracted
- » Insecure
- » Nervous anxiety
- » Scattered, panicky animals

Think 'Elemi' for:
Low immunity and animals that often have problems that arise quickly and then subside, especially if there is dry skin, breathing problems or erratic behaviour.
Stubborn skin conditions, that have no apparent cause, especially if the skin is dry and cracked.

EUCALYPTUS

(Eucalyptus Globulus, E. Radiata)

Element: Metal

History and Character
There are more than 300 varieties of eucalyptus tree, but most essential oil is distilled from the 'blue gum' tree, eucalyptus globulus. E.radiata is often preferred in aromatherapy because it has a sweeter fragrance and is less harsh on the skin, and safer for childre, having lower levels of 1.8 cineole, but it is not as powerful a disinfectant. I use both.

Eucalyptus are tall evergreen trees with greyish blue leaves that become yellow with age, and a pale trunk with strips of coloured bark that flakes off. Eucalyptus trees are native to Australia but have been introduced around the world. The eucalyptus tree draws up great quantities of water, drying out swamps so they can be farmed. The trees also release vapour loaded with the antiseptic essential oil, which repels malaria carrying mosquitoes that are often found in swampy areas. Traditionally the aborigines used eucalyptus to treat infections and fevers especially as a fumigant. Eucalyptus has a penetrating and drying energy, which dispels congestion of the lungs and lifts melancholy. It clears out frustrated energy and unconscious, stagnated feelings, allowing us to breathe freely, physically and emotionally. E.citriodora has similar uses but is more antifungal, bactericidal and insect repellent.

Synonyms
Gum Tree, Fever Tree, Stringy Bark.

Cultivation/sustainability
Widely cultivated. Eucalyptus plantations destroy native habitat in Europe. Prefer Australian oil.

Extraction and Characteristics
Steam distillation from fresh or part dried leaves and young twigs. The oil is a clear mobile liquid, yellowing with age.

Fragrance
Harshly camphoraceous, green, medicinal, with a slightly sweet undertone.

Principal Constituents
E.globulus
Oxides: 1,8 cineole
Terpenes: α-pinene, limonene, aromadendrene, ρ-cymene
Alcohols: globulol, trans-pinocarveol, ledol
Ketones: pinocarvone
Esters:α-terpenyl acetate
E.radiata
Terpenes: α-pinene, βpinene, myrcene
Alcohols: linalol, geraniol, α-terpineol, isoterpineol
Aldehydes: geranial, neral, citronellal, myrtenal

Actions
Antibacterial, anticatarrhal, antifungal, anti-inflammatory, antiseptic, antiviral, balsamic, decongestant, expectorant, insect repellent, mucolytic, rubefacient.

Safety

Externally non-toxic, non-irritant, (especially E.radiata), internally possibly toxic in amounts as small as 3.5 ml. E.globulus is contraindicated for the very young.

Principal Uses

Physical:
- » Asthma
- » Claustrophobia
- » Immunostimulant
- » Inhibition of viral activity, kills air-borne bacteria
- » Insect repellent
- » Respiratory decongestant
- » Thrush
- » Tight muscles

Behavioural:
- » Frustrated anger
- » Lack of will to participate in life's challenges
- » Those who feel frustrated by circumstance

Think 'Eucalyptus' for:

Animals who are frustrated in their environment, especially if this manifests as depression with angry outbursts.

Lung congestion, especially with excess mucous or high fever, or if the animal is run down.

FENNEL, SWEET

(Foeniculum Vulgare Var. Dulce)

Element: Earth (Metal)

History And Character

Fennel is a hardy perennial or biennial herb with soft, green, ferny leaves and umbrels of yellow flowers. Native to the shores of the Mediterranean it is now widely cultivated. Sweet or garden fennel is used in aromatherapy, not the bitter or common fennel, which has a high level of the potentially harmful ketone, fenchone. Traditionally, fennel has been used as a culinary herb worldwide. The Greeks used it as a diuretic to help them lose weight, and Ancient Olympic athletes ate it to promote strength. In Europe, fennel was hung over cottage doors as protection from witchcraft. It was known as an antidote to all sorts of poisons. Snakes were said to rub against it to improve their eyesight. Maybe because of its anti-toxic properties, fennel was said to give courage, strength and longevity. It is a warm, dry oil that has great affinity with the female reproductive system and the energy of nurture and care. It is good for those who over-think and worry about the welfare of others, or have an obsessive need to nurture (sometimes manifesting as phantom pregnancy), as it is helpful in finding ways to express a caring nature constructively. It also helps release gas and bloating in the digestive system, and generally relieves Dampness which can lead to fatty lumps and oedema.

Synonyms

F.officinale, F.capillaceum, Fenkel

Cultivation/sustainability

Cultivated

Fennel For Fatty lumps

A woman once called me seeking oils for her dog, who she described as an affectionate "dizzy blonde". In the course of the initial conversation, the woman said, "Really, I think it is me that needs the oils as much as her."

I find this is often the way, and was happy to work with someone who could acknowledge the symbiotic relationship we have with our animals when it comes to physical and emotional well-being. In this case I felt it would be particularly beneficial for them both to take oils as the human wanted to create a deeper connection with her dog. The woman had just had to make the awful decision to have her other dog put down. She described the dog who had passed on as her soulmate, but it was also the 'dizzy blondes' litter mate and both of them were missing her.

The dizzy blonde had also recently been diagnosed with cancerous mammary tumours so her person wanted oils that might help control progression of the disease, as well as cheer her up. The owner's issues were her grief at the loss of her other doggy companion and feeling that her energetic, emotional and spiritual boundaries were being disrespected in the home.

I gave both the dog and the woman bergamot (Citrus aurantium ssp.bergamia): uplifting, cleansing, anti-tumour, disperser of stagnant qi, encourages release of pent-up emotion, and helps us relax and let-go. They also needed Sweet fennel (Foeniculum vulgare var.dulce): releases stagnant qi in the stomach and intestines, has an affinity with the mammary glands, regulates hormone levels, encourages us to express ourselves and our creativity without fear, combats over-thinking and worry.

Even though the imbalances were apparently different, the same oils were good for both person and dog. It is as if the dog needed the oils on the physical level and the owner on the emotional level. In this case the oils had a positive effect on both owner and dog and the act of offering the oils helped them feel more connected.

Extraction and Characteristics
Steam distillation of the crushed seeds. The oil is a colourless to pale yellow liquid.

Fragrance
A sweet anise-like fragrance, sharp green with a warm earthy undertone.

Principal Constituents
Phenyl methyl ethers: trans-anethole, estragole
Terpenes: limonene, cis-ocimene, α-pinene, γ-terpinene, phellandrene, myrcene, terpinolene
Oxides: 1,8-cineole
Alcohols: fenchol
Ketones: fenchone

Actions
Analgesic, antibacterial, antifungal, anti-inflammatory, antiseptic, antispasmodic, cardiotonic, carminative, cholagogic, circulatory stimulant, decongestant, digestive, diuretic, emmenagogic, hormone-like, lactogenic, laxative, litholytic, oestrogen–like, respiratory tonic (rapid breathing).

Safety
Generally considered to be non-sensitising, but moderately irritating to the skin; use only in high dilutions. Do not use during pregnancy.

Principal Uses

Physical:
  - » Arthritis and similar conditions
  - » Constipation
  - » Fluid retention
  - » Intestinal gas
  - » Phantom pregnancy
  - » Poisonous bites
  - » Problems with lactation
  - » Respiratory distress
  - » Spasmodic colic
  - » To regulate hormonal cycles, unpredictable behaviour around seasons
  - » Urinary infections

Behavioural:
  - » Anxiety-related obsessive behaviours
  - » Over or under active nurture impulse
  - » Those who worry about others or seek constant reassurance

Think 'Sweet Fennel' for:
Emotionally insecure animals who are over-concerned with others, especially if there is a history of digestive upsets, flatulence, hormonal imbalance or fluid retention.
Obsessive anxiety.
Tumours and soft lumps, especially mammary.

FLOUVE

(Anthoxanthum Odoratum)

Element: Metal

History and Character

A tufted perennial grass with compact narrow leaves and dense compact flower spikes up to 3cm/1.5 ins long. Flouve is native to Europe, temperate Asia and Africa. The oil was out of favour for some years because in the 1950s, trials showed it caused liver cancer in mice due to its high levels of coumarin. However, recent trials have shown it to be safe for humans. In fact in recent trials on hospital patients in Ireland, coumarin was found to reduce tumours in cancer of the breast, skin and kidneys, and to boost the immune systems of patients with glandular fever and chronic fatigue syndrome. I have used it extensively for animals with allergies, especially pollen-based, irritated upper-respiratory tract, and head-shaking (a condition found in horses that can make them unrideable). I have also used it in the control of benign tumours and fatty lumps in dogs. Emotionally, flouve is drying and relieves irritation, giving inner space so there is no need for outer protectiveness. I use hay absolute, (same plant, different distillation method) interchangeably with flouve as both these oils can be hard to find.

Synonym

Sweet Vernal Grass.

Cultivation/sustainability

Cultivated

Extraction and Characteristics

Steam distillation of the grass heads. The oil has a dark brown viscous appearance.

Fragrance

Warm, sweet, honeyed, half-dry hay, with a dark spicy note.

Principal Constituents

Coumarin glycosides

Actions

Analgesic, antispasmodic, immunostimulant and stimulant.

Safety

Flouve can have quite high levels of coumarins, an anticoagulant so should not be used in conjunction with drugs such as Warfarin or Heparin.

Principal Uses

Physical:
  » Allergies
  » Chronic illnesses
  » Compromised immune systems
  » Cushing's syndrome
  » Fatty lumps
  » Head-shaking
  » Sinus problems
  » Tumours

Behavioural:
  » Aloof
  » Despairing
  » Shut down

Think 'Flouve' for:

Allergies, especially if the animal seems remote or disengaged.

Animals who seem to succumb easily to illness, especially if they display symptoms of allergic reactions.

Tumours.

FRANKINCENSE

(Boswellia sacra/carterii)

Element: Earth (Metal)

History and Character

Frankincense is a small tree or shrub with masses of pinnate leaves and white or pale-pink flowers. It grows wild throughout the deserts of North-East Africa. It has been an important incense in all the religions of the world since the Ancient Egyptians. Frankincense slows and deepens breathing, which is why frankincense is useful for asthma. It is also said to "distance the mind from worries and fears". Frankincense eases the passage into death and can be used when trying to decide whether to euthanize an animal. Frankincense also helps us let go of the past and old attachments that have outgrown their usefulness. It calms and centres the mind, allowing us to focus on the present. Due to overharvesting to fulfill the demand for essential oil the wild population is suffering.

Synonyms

Olibanum, Gum Rhus.

Cultivation/sustainability

Wildcrafted. Near threatened status, very important to find sustainable sources when buying.

Extraction and Characteristics

Steam distillation from the oleo gum resin. It is a pale yellowish to green liquid.

Frankincense eases Ghost's transition

One autumn I arrived at my friend Wendy Wolfe's house to teach a workshop, to find that her beloved 18-year-old goat, Ghost, was not well. He had been failing all summer and we knew he was preparing to leave, but now he lay down all the time, hardly eating, and was uncomfortably constipated. Wendy had called the vet to come the next morning to put him down, but she was not completely at peace with the decision.

It is always hard to separate between our own emotion about letting go of animal friends and their own needs and wishes. We have the power of life over death and sometimes in our wish "to do the right thing" and end what we perceive to be suffering, we speed up a process which has its own mystery and takes it own time, this is where frankincense helps us. Offer your animal frankincense and it will become clear.

That evening we went out to visit Ghost and took a bottle of frankincense with us. He was lying down quietly when we walked into his pen but looked at us softly. I held the open bottle of frankincense about 30cm/12 ins from his nose and watched keenly for his response. I did not want to force him to stand if he wanted to distance himself from the fragrance, so I was prepared to move away quickly, if necessary. However, Ghost sniffed strongly and moved his head towards the bottle, so I moved the bottle closer to him. He breathed deeply for a minute or so, going into a trance, then stood up and defecated for the first time in two days. I gave him a few more sniffs and he moved his body into my hand so I rubbed a little oil into the association point for his Stomach meridian. He then wandered over to his hay pile and nibbled at it. We left him, hoping his last night would be a peaceful one.

The next morning Wendy went down to have a few last words with him before the vet arrived, only to find him up, eating, and in no mood to leave this world yet. Wendy cancelled the vet. The week of the course was a wonderful sunny September and Ghost enjoyed every moment, he scrambled around his rocky paddock taking in the sun, ate well, and seemed to have normal bowel movements. He was drinking a small amount of peppermint hydrosol daily (15 ml/1 tbsp in a bucket of water) and had a small sniff of frankincense each day. He interacted with the students, touching everyone with his wisdom and kindness, and received a lot of love and attention from us all during the week-long course.

I returned to the UK at the end of the week. When I arrived home I found a message from Wendy that Ghost had died peacefully in the night as I was flying across the Atlantic. Frankincense allows our animals to release from their bodies peacefully, and gives us the space to allow it to happen.

Fragrance
Sweet, balsamic top-note and resinous, smoky bottom-note.

Principal Constituents
Esters: octyl acetate, incensyl acetate, bornyl acetate
Alcohols: octanol, incensol, linalol
Terpenes: sabinene, α-pinene, limonene, α-thujene, ρ-cymene

Actions
Analgesic, anticatarrhal, anti-depressive, anti-inflammatory, antiseptic, antioxidant, cicatrisant, energising, expectorant, immunostimulant.

Safety
Generally held to be non-toxic, non-irritant and non-sensitising.

Principal Uses

Physical:
>> Asthma
>> Claustrophobia
>> Diarrhoea, especially if triggered by nerves
>> Scars, ulcers and wounds
>> To ease the passage into death

Behavioural:
>> Anxiety and restlessness
>> Noise sensitivity
>> Specific fears, e.g. fireworks
>> Stereo-typical behaviours (cribbing, pacing, spinning)

Think 'Frankincense' for:
Anxious or fearful animals, especially if there are signs of claustrophobia such as pacing or refusing to go into enclosed areas, or asthma, or loose stools.
Fear of fireworks and other known triggers.
When deciding about euthanasia.

GARLIC

(Allium Sativum)

Element: Metal (Fire)

History and character

Most of us know what a garlic bulb looks like, a strong white skin surrounding a cluster of 'teeth' or cloves that are succulent and pungent. Garlic has been considered a cure-all for millennia, the Pyramid builders ate it to give them strength and it is still used by all three classical healing systems: Traditional Chinese Medicine, Ayurvedic medicine, and European medicine. In the first century BC, the Greek physician Dioscorides stated that garlic "clears the arteries and opens the mouth of the veins". Garlic was a 'tool of magic power' for traditional medicine men, and science has now proved that garlic is a powerful natural antibiotic. It also reduces blood pressure and stimulates T-cells. Energetically, it burns through blockages, clearing the way for healing.

Synonyms

Poor Man's Treacle, Allium.

Cultivation/sustainability

Cultivated

Extraction and characteristics

The essential oil is extracted by steam distillation from the fresh, crushed bulbs.

Fragrance

Sharp, pungent, sweet.

Principal constituents

Organic Sulphides: diallyl disulphide, di-2-propenyl-trisulphide,3'-thiobis-1-propene, diallyl tetrasulphide
Alcohols: methyl 2-propenyl-disulphide, Methyl 2-propenyl-trisulphide

Actions

Anthelmintic, antibiotic, antibacterial, antimicrobial, antiseptic, antifungal, antiviral, anti-toxic, antioxidant, antispasmodic, decongestant, expectorant, hypotensive, immunostimulant, parasiticide, vasodilator.   .

Safety

Generally non-toxic, but dermal irritant so dilute well, do not use on hypersensitive, diseased, or damaged skin. When applying to skin always add equal parts chamomile (German) or yarrow to counteract harshness. Garlic inhibits blood clotting and should not be used with other blood thinning medicine such as Warfarin, Heparin, or aspirin. Over use of garlic (the plant) can cause anaemia in dogs and horses.

Principal uses
Physical:
- » Abscesses
- » Bronchitis
- » Catarrh
- » Infected wounds
- » Influenza
- » Intestinal parasites
- » Kennel cough
- » Laminitis
- » Lung infections
- » Lung worm
- » Mange
- » Mites
- » Mud fever
- » Navicular

Think 'Garlic' for:
All infectious diseases and infected wounds, if there is a lot of pus or mucous present. Animals debilitated by neglect.

GERANIUM

(Pelargonium Graveolens)

Element: Water (Fire)

History and Character
A sprawling, aromatic perennial shrub with hairy serrated leaves and small pink flowers. Pelargonium graveolens is native to South Africa but widely cultivated. Until recently, essential oil was mostly produced in Reunion (Bourbon), Egypt, Madagascar and China, with the Bourbon oil being the most prized; South Africa now produces a very good quality oil as well. Because there is so much confusion between pelargonium, which we call geranium, and true geranium, which we call cranesbill or herb Robert, it is unclear what the historical uses of the plant are. Nonetheless, the strongest physical and energetic action of geranium oil is 'to regulate'. This is due to its powerful effect on the adrenal cortex, which regulates hormones and other endocrine functions. It is one of the most Yin of the essential oils and helps us to reconnect with the feminine principle within ourselves, increasing sensitivity, spontaneity, and our ability to receive making us feel secure in ourselves. Geranium can be used anywhere there is a lack of Yin, which is characterised by dryness rigidity, or over-heating, and is especially good for mature females.

Synonyms
Rose Geranium, Pelargonium.

Pelargonia, the geranium cat

Pelargonia was a 15-year old cat who, with her people, had recently moved house. Once a brave cat who was mostly outside, she had become timid and withdrawn, avoiding physical contact, sleeping a lot and seeming depressed. Her skin was dry and flaky and her coat rather dull. I offered her geranium hydrosol which was indicated because she is an older cat with flaky skin, has recently moved, and because of her name!

After initial interest, Pelargonia was reticent about taking the hydrosol, so I suggested her person add a few drops to a saucer of water and leave them where she could self-medicate privately (cats can be a bit cagey, as we know!) but not in a place she would normally go to.

Over the next few days, Pelargonia was observed sleeping curled up near the saucer a few times throughout the day. On the third day, she came to her owner, made her sit down and have a cuddle, then got up stretched and went outside. From then on her confidence returned and her coat improved.

Cultivation/sustainability
Cultivated

Extraction and Characteristics
Steam distillation of the leaves, stalks and flowers. The oil is a wonderful clear green colour.

Fragrance
A very sweet and fresh, slightly spicy top-note, with green mid-notes and a musty, river-bottom, bottom-note.

Principal Constituents
Alcohols: citronellol, geraniol, linalol
Esters: citronellyl formate, geranyl formate, geranyl tiglate
Aldehydes: geranial, citronellal
Ketones: isomenthone, menthone

Actions
Analgesic, antibacterial, antidiabetic, antifungal, anti-inflammatory, antiseptic, antispasmodic, astringent, cicatrisant, decongestant, digestive, haemostatic, insect repellent, phlebotonic (lymph) relaxant, tonic to liver and kidneys.

Safety

Generally held to be non-toxic, non-irritant and non-sensitising; dermatitis has been seen in some individuals, especially with the Bourbon type.

Principal Uses

Physical
- » Hormone problems
- » Skin problems, especially greasy dandruff
- » Lice and mosquitoes
- » Fungal infections of the skin
- » Dry or greasy flaky skin
- » Facial neuralgia

Behavioural
- » Insecure, moody types
- » New home or other disruptions to lifestyle

Think 'Geranium' for:

Insecure or depressed animals who lack self-confidence, especially if their moods are cyclical or their skin is over dry, greasy or unbalanced.

Older females/adolescent males who show a lack of receptivity.

GINGER

(Zingiber Officinale)

Element: Fire (Water)

History and Character

An erect, reed-like perennial herb growing from a spreading tuberous pungent rhizome, native to southern Asia but widely cultivated throughout the tropics. Ginger is a well-known cooking spice and healing remedy that has been used for thousands of years. Best known as a digestive, it is also used for nausea and travel sickness. Ginger is useful for all Excess Damp conditions e.g. overproduction of mucous, or diarrhoea. Because of its deeply warming nature, ginger is often appreciated by older animals and those who suffer from arthritis. Energetically, ginger is hot and stimulant and a restorative of Yang energy, giving a boost to those who lack physical energy. It also has a strong effect on what the Chinese call the Will, the personal drive to make a mark on the world (a function of the Water element). Ginger ignites those who lack confidence and the determination to carry things through, increases feelings of self-worth, and lifts despondency.

Synonyms

Common Ginger, Jamaican Ginger. There is also a related plant, Alphina Officinarum, known as Chinese Ginger

Cultivation/sustainability
Cultivated

Extraction and Characteristics
Steam distillation from the unpeeled, dried root. The oil is pale-yellow to amber liquid.

Fragrance
Warm, spicy, slightly earthy, pungent.

Principal Constituents
Terpenes: zingiberene, ar-curcumene, α-farnesene, ρ-cymene, β-sesquiphellandrene, camphene, bisabolene, α-pinene, α-phellandrene, limonene, β-pinene
Alcohols: nerolidol, 2-nonanol, citronellol, linalol, borneol
Oxides: 1,8 cineole

Actions
Analgesic, anticatarrhal, carminative, digestive, expectorant, general tonic, sexual tonic, stomachic.

Safety
Generally held to be non-toxic, non-irritant, possible sensitization.

Principal Uses

Physical:
  » Sluggish digestion
  » Flatulence
  » Diarrhoea
  » Soft lumps on skin
  » Arthritis
  » Pancreatic problems
  » Muscular aches and pains

  » Back ache
  » Congested lungs and sinus (white or clear mucous)
  » Lack of sexual performance
  » Travel sickness

Behavioural:
  » Lack of confidence
  » Depression

Think 'Ginger' for:
Depressed, run down animals, especially if they have non-specific skin nodules or other symptoms of Excess Damp such as diarrhoea or clear mucous.
Old animals that feel the cold and may be stiff.

GRAPEFRUIT

(Citrus X Paradisii)

Element: Wood (Earth)

History and Character
A large citrus tree, with glossy green leaves and large yellow fruits. It is native to tropical Asia but cultivated in California, Florida, Brazil and Israel. It is a recent hybrid but shares the high vitamin C levels of other citrus fruits and is also said to help with lymphatic drainage. Energetically, it is cleansing and uplifting, dispelling blockages that lead to frustration and irritability. It breaks down and facilitates absorption of fat, and helps in the assimilation of emotional changes.

Synonyms
C. Racemosa.

Extraction and Characteristics
Cold-pressed from the fresh peel the oil is a yellowish green liquid. There is also an oil steam distilled from the whole fruit but this is inferior.

Cultivation/sustainability
Cultivated. Use only organic

Fragrance
Fresh, light, fruity and slightly bitter.

Principal Constituents
Terpenes: limonene, myrcene
Aldehydes: octanal, decanal
Ketones: nootketone
Alcohols and esters are present in large numbers but in individually low amounts. The characteristic aroma of grapefruit is due to the sesquiterpene nootketone.

Actions
Antiseptic, antibacterial, astringent, carminative, digestive, diuretic, immune stimulant, tonic.

Safety
Generally held to be non-toxic, non-irritant and non-sensitising, however it contains low levels of coumarins, so could be photo-toxic. The suggested use is no higher than 4% dilution on skin exposed to ultraviolet light.

Grapefruit and Ginger for a smooth journey

Courtesy of Sarah Loveridge, Level 2 Animal PsychAromatica student

Tina, a mixed breed female dog, is a much loved family pet, fat and friendly with a penchant for biscuits. However, when Tina rides in the car, she pants heavily and noisily and salivates a lot. Previously, she was afraid to get into the car, but now she wants to go out in the car until the engine is started, then the panting starts. She also nibbles trouser legs when people arrive at the house.

Tina is fed a low-quality commercial dog food, is overweight and under-exercised, all of these things could make her feel nauseous when in the car. Also, Tina is very much "in charge" at home, ushering in guests, sleeping wherever she wants, and demanding food and attention. This means her stress levels are high and strengthens the feeling of being out of control when she is in the car.

Tina's people were asked to try and help reduce her feelings of responsibility through simple rules that make it clear to Tina that she is lower in the pack than her people. For example, by asking her to 'work for food' or any other benefits, such as sofa time, this simply meant she had to sit whenever she wanted something.

Tina was offered ginger essential oil, a classic remedy for car sickness, it also stimulates digestion and circulation, and helps build confidence; and grapefruit essential oil, which aids digestion, stimulates break down of fats, is uplifting, and helps refresh the mind. Tina licked the oils enthusiastically for six days, then started to lose interest, by day eight she refused the grapefruit and on the tenth day she was finished with the oils. On day three of the treatment, Tina went out in the car and was much calmer.

At day 10 her people reported, "Tina seems to be a much happier dog since we decided to take charge of her behaviour, she doesn't seem to mind us being more strict with her. She learned quickly that if she wants something she has to sit. She is also doing less trouser nibbling, as most of the time she is asked to sit while people come in. Tina is a new dog in the car. Sometimes, we hardly know she's there!"

Principal Uses

Physical:
- » To stimulate lymphatic drainage and digestion
- » To cleanse the liver and gallbladder
- » Muscle fatigue (with juniper berry)
- » Overeating/food obsessive
- » Irritable bowels
- » Colitis

Behavioural:
- » Depression
- » Confusion
- » Irritability

Think 'Grapefruit' for:

When there is a recurrence of minor illnesses, especially if the animal is irritable or lethargic and there is a tendency to carry excess weight.

As a supporting oil to other Liver/anger cleansing oils.

Long-running digestive disturbances especially if accompanied by anxiety or lymphatic congestion.

HELICHRYSUM

(Helichrysum Italicum)

Element: Wood (Metal)

History and Character

A strongly aromatic shrub, about 60 cm/2ft high with a multi-branched stem of silvery, lanceolate leaves, native to the Mediterranean (especially the east). The small, bright yellow, daisy-like flowers become dry as the plant matures but still retain their colour and fragrance, hence the common name of everlast or immortelle. Traditionally used in a decoction for migraine, chronic respiratory problems, liver ailments and all types of skin conditions, this is the best essential oil for bruises. You can practically watch the bruise fade before your eyes after applying a few drops of undiluted helichrysum, plus, unlike the other famous bruise remedy, arnica, it can be used on broken skin to disinfect cuts. Helichrysum has a similar effect on bruised emotions, dissolving resentment held over from past hurt. Energetically, helichrysum releases blocked energy, especially anger that has been repressed and become simmering and resentful.

Synonyms

Everlast, Immortelle, St John's Herb.

Cultivation/sustainability

Cultivated sources available. Some danger of over-harvesting wild plants.

Helichrysum for a Hen in a crisis

Courtesy of Mary Lindo, VN, mGEOTA

Doris had been attacked by a fox and left with severe muscle lacerations on her back. The fox had also killed one of her companions. Although she survived and had been treated by her vet with antibiotics and painkillers, Doris simply lay on her nest, not moving, eating or drinking.

Doris selected: Helichrysum (Helichrysum italicum ssp serotinum), for brusing and trauma; Neroli (Citrus aurantium var bigarade), uplifting and comforting, useful for states of shock and animals that have lost the will to live; seaweed, (fucus vesiculosa) a powerful immune stimulant, strengthening resistance to disease and recovery from infection. Each diluted 1 drop in 10 ml sunflower oil.

The first evening Doris was offered the oils she reacted the same way to each oil. She closed her eyes and rested her beak on the bottle, having to be gently removed after a few minutes. That night she laid an egg. Thursday morning she again reacted to all the oils dilating her eyes and breathing them in deeply for several minutes, going into a trance and needing to be gently removed. That evening her reactions to the oils were slightly different: Helichrysum: eyes dilated, stuck beak in bottle and rested there for a few minutes; Neroli, eyes dilated and breathed the aroma in deeply for seven/eight seconds; Seaweed closed eyes and turned away.

Saturday morning she turned away from the oils and started walking away, although still limping badly. By the end of the day she was drinking for herself and starting to peck around and showed no further interest in the oils.

Extraction and Characteristics

Steam distillation from the fresh flowers. It is a pale yellow, red-tinged oil with a powerful honey-like scent and a slightly bitter/pungent undertone.

Principal Constituents

Esters: neryl acetate, neryl butyrate
Ketones: beta-diones
Alcohols: nerol, geraniol, linalol
Terpenes: limonene, pinene, beta-caryophyllene
Aldehydes: isovaleric
Phenols: eugenol

Actions

Anti-allergenic, anticatarrhal, anticoagulant, antidiabetic, antifungal, antihaematomic, anti-inflammatory, antiseptic, antispasmodic, antiviral, digestive, cholagogic, cicatrizant, hepatic, mucolytic, neurotonic, phlebotonic, stimulant.

Safety

Generally held to be non-toxic, non-irritant and non-sensitising.

Principal Uses

Physical:
  » Bruises and wounds
  » Nervous exhaustion
  » Allergies
  » Burns, boils, eczema
  » Hepatic congestion
  » Aches, pains, strains
  » Asthma, bronchitis, chronic coughs
  » Bacterial infections

Behavioural:
  » Deeply bruised emotions
  » Habitually negative behaviour
  » Past abuse
  » Resentful, simmering anger

Think "Helichrysum" for:

Animals that are holding resentment over past treatment and are stuck in negative patterns that are no longer useful, especially if they have irritated skin.
Any bumps/bruises, impact injury, rash, or burn.

HEMP

(Cannabis x Sativa L)

Element: Wood (Fire)

History and Character:

Hemp is an annual plant that grows up to 4 metres/12 ft high with characteristic sharp-tipped leaves. Native to Asia, it can grow in most temperate climates and is cultivated worldwide, both illicitly for the drug trade and legally for the production of fibres. The drug is mentioned in early Hindu and Chinese works on medicine. The Hindus use it as a digestive aid and as part of spiritual practice in the worship of Shiva, god of destruction and regeneration. Its use slowly spread through Persia to the Arabs, where it was used by the Mohammedan sect known as Hashishin or assassins. From here cannabis was introduced to the Crusaders in the 11th/12th centuries. Hemp has been used medicinally as a relaxant, for the control of nausea, and as a general antispasmodic. Energetically, hemp is warming, putting fire in the belly, and euphoric, lifting you above the physical body and worldly cares. Used in moderation it releases blocked energy, and helps an animal reconnect to its essential nature, giving increased energy and optimism.

Synonyms
Marijuana, Grass.

Cultivation/sustainability
Cultivated. Least concern

Extraction and Characteristics
Steam distillation from leaves and flowering tops. It is slightly viscous with a pale golden yellow colour.

Fragrance
Warm, earthy, herbaceous, slightly sweet, with a spicy undertone.

Principal Constituents
Ketones: isopinocamphone, pinocamphone
Terpenes: beta pinene, germacrene D, elixine, aromadendrene caryophollene, beta bourbonene, humulene
Alcohols: elemol, myrtenol

Actions
Analgesic, anxiolytic, anticonvulsant, antiemetic, antispasmodic, antitussive, cicatrisant, muscle relaxant, possibly hormonal adaptogen, soporific.

Safety
Caution with epilepsy, dilute well, use in moderation.

Principal Uses
Physical:
- » Nausea
- » Muscle fatigue and cramps
- » Respiratory tightness
- » Hormonal imbalances
- » Spasms of any sort
- » Glaucoma

Behavioural:
- » Hyperactivity
- » Separation anxiety
- » Insecurity
- » Easily overwhelmed
- » Restless anxiety
- » Apathy
- » Obsessive behaviours

Think 'Hemp' for:
Animals who show anxious obsessive behaviours, especially if they have digestive problems or show excessive or insufficient appetite, or are intolerant of others, or have gone through recent upheavals.
Older animals who suffer from the cold and restless, anxious behaviour.

HYSSOP

(Hyssopus Officinalis Var Decumbens)

Element: Metal

History and Character:

Hyssop is a small shrub with glossy, green leaves and spires of blue flowers. Native to the Mediterranean it is now widely cultivated and grows wild throughout temperate climates. The Hebrews used it to purify the temples and it is mentioned in the Old Testament as Ezob. The Romans used it for protection against plague; in fact, protection is a theme with hyssop as you will see. For the body, hyssop has traditionally been used for upper respiratory infections and fevers; also for indigestion particularly abdominal bloating. Hyssop has a hot, drying energy and is very assertive, invigorating body, mind and spirit, and helping to 'pull everything together'. Hyssop makes animals feel secure within their own physical and energetic boundaries so outside influences can no longer disturb them, particularly the moods of others.

Synonyms

Azob, not to be confused with Hedge Hyssop (Gratiola officinalis).

Cultivation/sustainability

Cultivated or wildcrafted. No concerns

Extraction and Characteristics

Steam distillation from leaves and flowering tops. Pale yellow/green liquid.

Fragrance

Pungent, camphoraceous, sweet, herbaceous, warm and spicy.

Principal Constituents

Terpenes: α-thujene, α-pinene, sabinene, β-pinene, β-trans-ocimene, p-cymene, limonene
Oxides: eucalyptol
Alcohols: α-pinocarveol, α-terpineol
Acetates: myrtenal
Ketones: pinocarvone, isapinocamphone

Actions

Antibacterial, antirheumatic, antispasmodic, antiviral, astringent, cicatrisant, decongestant, digestive, diuretic, expectorant, hypertensive, immune tonic, litholytic, sudorific, tonic (circulation, general, heart), vermifuge, vulnerary.

Safety

Avoid use in epilepsy; do not use in fever; do not use in pregnancy or young animals. Dilute well, use in moderation. There are four chemotypes of H.officinalis, var decumbens is the safest to use.

Principal Uses

Physical:

- » Breathlessness
- » Immune deficiency
- » Bloating
- » Appetite loss
- » Infections of the respiratory tract
- » Rheumatism

Behavioural:

- » Obsessive behaviours
- » Melancholy, despair
- » Lack of personal boundaries, physically and emotionally

Think 'Hyssop' for:

Animals who are oversensitive to the moods of those around them, or easily upset by their environment, especially if they are prone to respiratory problems.

Defensive aggression and other situations where personal boundaries are an issue.

JASMINE

(Jasminum Officinale)

Element: Fire (Water)

History and Character:

The star-shaped, waxy jasmine flower grows on an evergreen vine or shrub. It is native to China, northern India and west Asia and there are many varieties. The fragrance of jasmine is considered to be one of the most sensually evocative and is strongest after dark and just before dawn, which is when the flowers are harvested for oil production. Because the flowers are so delicate they must be harvested by hand, yielding only a little essential oil which is hard to extract apart from as an absolute. For this reason jasmine is an expensive item, but is indispensable in its role as a Yang balancer. Traditionally jasmine was known as a fertility herb and has been used as an aphrodisiac and to facilitate birth. It is a warming, euphoric oil that instils optimism, eases nervous anxiety, and soothes restlessness. In aromatherapy, it is known as 'King of oils' as, despite its sweet, floral top-note, it has a particular affinity with male hormonal and excess Yang behaviours, especially for males who act 'macho' to hide insecurity.

Synonyms

Jasmin, Jessamine, Common Jasmine.

Jasmine for the reluctant leader

Jermaine was a 10 year old Hanoverian gelding. He was a big boy and the star of the riding stable, competing to an advanced level in dressage. However, he had a tendency to throw his weight around, bullying the smaller horses in the field where he was turned out and walking over people who tried to handle him. He was not bad-natured; in fact, he was a big softy who felt overwhelmed by his responsibilities as leader of the herd, so had to enforce his position through aggression. I offered him jasmine diluted 3 drops to 5 ml in sunflower oil. Jermaine showed keen interest in the oil, sniffing and licking for 3 days, by which time there was an obvious change in his behaviour. He seemed much more respectful of the humans who handled him, more relaxed and happier in himself, and the worry lines around his eyes disappeared. He showed mild interest for the next 2 days, then lost interest completely, at which stage he was noticeably calmer and less aggressive in the field and even allowed other horses to eat with him.

Cultivation/sustainability
Cultivated

Extraction and Characteristics
Jasmine is usually found as an absolute, from solvent extracted concrete. An essential oil is sometimes made by steam distillation of the absolute. The absolute is a thick orangey liquid.

Fragrance
An intensely sweet, floral top-note with a musky bottom-note.

Principal Constituents
Esters: benzyl acetate, benzyl benzoate, phytyl acetate, methyl linoleate, methyl jasmonate
Alcohols: linalol, phytol, isophytol, geraniol, benzyl alcohol
Ketones: cis-jasmone
Imines: indole
Phenols: eugenol

Actions
Analgesic, antidepressant, calmative, carminative, cicatrisant, emollient, sexual tonic, uterine tonic.

Safety
Generally held to be non-toxic, non-irritant and non-sensitising. Allergic reactions have been seen in some individuals. It is sometimes contaminated with the solvent hexane, used to separate the absolute from the concrete.

Principal Uses

Physical:
- » Infertility
- » Impotence

Behavioural:
- » Sexual anxiety
- » Nervous anxiety
- » Headstrong
- » Bullying
- » Insecurity
- » Excess 'Yang' behaviour
- » Pushy 'take control' types

Think 'Jasmine' for:

Bullying or other hierarchy issues, especially if the animal has been left in a position of responsibility that it does not feel up to, and is nervous when separated from others.

Animals who want to take charge in a forceful manner because they are actually insecure.

JUNIPER BERRY

(Juniperus Communis)

Element: Water (Metal)

History and Character

A shrubby, evergreen tree with bluish green needles, small flowers and green or black berries, juniper is found throughout the northern hemisphere. There are several species of juniper from which an oil is produced and their actions are different, so pay attention to the Latin name. Traditionally juniper berry has been used for urinary infections, respiratory problems and gastro-intestinal conditions; it also flushes out the liver and breaks down uric acid. Juniper's sharp pungent fragrance dispels negativity and since ancient times it has been used for spiritual purification; it is especially powerful at clearing out and protecting our psychic space. Juniper benefits those who are overwhelmed by crowds, or lack confidence in social groups, and helps to settle those who feel restless after being at 'an occasion'.

Synonyms

Common Juniper

Cultivation/sustainability

Cultivated or wildcrafted. No concerns

Extraction and Characteristics

Steam distillation of the fresh berries, sometimes fermented berries are used, this is an inferior product. There is also an inferior oil made from the twigs and wood. The oil is a clear or slightly yellow mobile liquid.

Fragrance
Camphoraceous, fresh, piney, with a warm, woody undertone.

Principal Constituents
Terpenes: α-pinene, limonene, β-pinene, myrcene, sabinene, τ-terpinene, α-thujene, δ-cadinene, ρ-cymene, α-terpinene, β-caryophyllene, terpinolene
Alcohols:terpinen-4-ol

Actions
Analgesic, anti-diabetic, antiseptic, detoxicant, digestive tonic, diuretic, hypo-uricemic (breaks down uric acid), litholytic, soporific.

Safety
Generally held to be non-toxic, non-irritant and non-sensitising. It should be used with caution in patients with kidney inflammation as high levels of the diuretics 4-terpineol and terpinen-4-ol may cause irritation. Do not use in pregnancy.

Principal Uses

Physical:
  » Arthritis
  » Oedema
  » Overworked soft tissue
  » Muscle cramps
  » Kidney infection
  » After medical procedures to cleanse the liver

Behavioural:
  » Restlessness
  » Suspicion
  » Those who are overwhelmed by or restless in crowds
  » Nervous snappishness

Think 'juniper berry' for:
Animals who have withdrawn into themselves, often being grumpy and actively protective of their space, especially if there is any stiffness of joints or muscles or a weakening of the bladder, or there is a history of medical procedures that required anaesthetic.
Those who fall apart in crowds becoming fearful and withdrawn.

LAVENDER

(Lavandula Angustifolia/Officinalis)

Element: Fire (Wood)

History and Character

An evergreen perennial herb, with pale spiky leaves and violet blue flowers that rise above the main bush on slender stalks. Native to the Mediterranean but now cultivated all over the world, traditionally the best oil came from Provence in France. Lavender has a wide range of uses and has been with us as a folk remedy for a long, long, time. It is a cure-all and intimately linked with the development of aromatherapy as we know it today. Lavender is said to have a highly synergistic nature, strengthening the actions of other oils it is blended with. Energetically lavender is cool and dry, soothing our brows in times of feverish emotions. It stills the heart and helps oversensitive individuals to express themselves freely. It is particularly useful for those whose emotions overwhelm reason, paralysing action or inducing hysteria. Many countries produce good quality lavender now, and it is worth having a selection as each lavender carries the energy of the land and culture that produced it. Lavender from England is genteel, moist and very soothing, lavender from Israel is hot, dry and very fast-acting; lavender grown at high altitude is the most energetically refined. I call lavender Florence Nightingale, after the famous British nurse, because you can always call on her for a little light nursing or when in need of extra TLC, either physically or emotionally.

Synonyms

Vera, Common Lavender, Garden Lavender.

Cultivation/sustainability

Widely cultivated. Always prefer organic

Extraction and Characteristics

Steam distillation of the fresh flowering tops.

Fragrance

Sweet, herbaceous, floral, slightly camphoraceous.

Principal Constituents

Esters: linalyl acetate, lavandulyl acetate

Alcohols: linalol, terpinen-4-ol, lavandulol
Terpenes: cis-caryophyllene, limonene, β-caryophyllene
Oxides: 1,8 cineole

Actions

Analgesic, antibacterial, antifungal, anti-inflammatory, antiseptic, antispasmodic, calmative, cardiotonic, carminative, cicatrisant, emmenagogic, hypotensive, sedative, tonic.

Lavender sets things right

Proud flesh is the overdevelopment of tissue around a healing wound, caused by excessive granulation. This is a common problem and I have many case studies, one of my most recent was an older riding-school horse, who was forced into retirement by a large wound near her front knee that had chronic proud flesh. The wound had not healed in eight months. With her permission, I applied a solution of lavender in calendula oil and after three weeks the proud flesh had dramatically reduced, and the wound went on to heal completely by the end of five weeks. The horse was also offered lavender oil to inhale at the same time, which lifted her spirits and helped her relax in her new lifestyle.

Safety

Generally held to be non-toxic, non-irritant and non-sensitising. May be applied to the skin without dilution, however lavender oil is often adulterated.

Principal Uses

Physical:
  » Stress-related skin conditions
  » Burns
  » Scars
  » Wounds
  » Proud flesh
  » Swellings
  » Sinusitis
  » Flea repellent
  » To support other oils

Behavioural:
  » Nervous hysteria
  » Shyness
  » Shock

Think 'Lavender' for:

All skin conditions, especially especially burns and proud flesh and if the animal has a strong need for connection, or shows nervous restlessness.
Shy, timid animals who want to connect but don't dare.

LAVENDER GREEN

(Lavandula viridis)

History and Character:

Lavandula viridis, commonly known as green lavender or white lavender, is a species of flowering plant in the family Lamiaceae, occurring naturally in Spain and Portugal. The plant is very distinctive and intriguing, with pale yellow/green stamens and softer, greener leaves than "normal" lavender. It is comparatively rare, growing in distinct patches in the damper folds of the dry hills, between its purple relatives Lavandula stoechas.

A research study published in 2011 in the Journal of Medical Microbiology identified fifty-one essential oil compounds in this species. Among the fifty-one compounds, 1,8-cineole, camphor, alpha-pinene, and linalool had the highest percentages, respectively. From these results we can see how the essential oil is anti-infectious and opens the lungs, and is at the same time soothing and gentle.

I have included this oil because of its powerful anti-fungal activity. Research has found that the essential oil has a strong antifungal activity against yeasts and filamentous fungi, specifically strains of Candida, Aspergillus, Trichophyton, Epidermophyton, and Cryptococcus.

Energetically, green lavender has a soft, moist, yin supportive effect, giving a feeling of "I can do it". It is relaxing and stimulating, allowing clarity of purpose and lightness of heart.

Synonyms

White lavender, Lavandula massonii, Lavandula Stoechas var. albiflora

Cultivation/sustainability

Wildcrafted, no issues.

Extraction and Characteristics:

Steam distillation of flowering stems. A clear to pale yellow, mobile liquid

Fragrance

Green, camphoraceous, fresh, lemon

Principal Constituents

1.8-cineole, camphor, alpha-pinene, borneol, beta-pinene, delta 3-carene, alpha-terpineol, linalool

Safety

Dilute well for use, especially with youngsters.

Principal uses

Physical:
  » Fungal infections
  » Mud fever
  » Sinusitis,
  » Moist coughs

Behavioural:
  » Lack of confidence
  » Easily overwhelmed
  » Frozen emotions
  » Anxiety

Think "Green lavender"

Those who feel easily overwhelmed by taking care, especially animals prone to fungal infections or excess mucous.

All fungal infections

LENTISK

(Pistacia lentiscus)

Element: Metal

History and Character

Commonly known as mastic or lentisk, this large shrub/small tree is widespread around the Mediterranean basin, Iberian peninsula and most famously Crete. The plant flowers in spring with peculiar small deeply red flowers, which contrast with the deep green of its leaves. All parts of the bush are aromatic. The pea-sized red berries are edible, but only appear on the female plant. The shrubs grow on wild, rocky, sun-exposed hillsides, by preference. The species is important, from an ecological point of view, to the recovery and evolution of degraded areas. The essential oil is steam distilled from the leaves and twigs (and occasionally berries or flowers) and properly is known as Lentisk. Mastic is the gum collected by making incisions in the stem. This can also be distilled for essential oil.

Many ancient writers refer to the lentisk or mastic bush. Dioscurides, in his De Materia Medica (ca 70AD), tells us that 'Schinos is a well known tree, all its parts are warming and astringent, the fruit as well as the leaves and the bark have the same properties. A decoction of these parts is astringent and beneficial for dysenteri, diarrhea and stomach bleeding ... as a mouthwash it 'rescues loose teeth'..and it 'cleans the face and gives it a healthy colour'. It was the orginal chewing gum and is still considered beneficial for gum health, reducing plaque. It's also traditionally used for coughs and bronchitis, and as a treatment for diarrhoea. Externally it is applied to boils, ulcers, ringworm and muscular stiffness.

Today, many of mastic's traditional uses are confirmed, including its beneficial effect on oral health and digestive function, although most of the studies were carried out with the gum. It has also shown some action against cancer cells in-vitro.

It carries the energy of wild hills and energetically gives a feeling of spaciousness, reconnecting you to your instinctive soul (Po) and sharpening the senses. It helps to reset the mental/

emotional terrain for a new outlook on life, bringing an inner relaxation and a feeling of optimism, for those who are "hanging on by a thread". This is helpful for animals who need to move on from past bad experiences, especially if they have been enclosed against their will.

Synonyms
Mastic tree, wild pistachio, tears of chios, Lentiscus massiliensis, Terebinthus lentiscus

Extraction and Characteristics
Steam distillation of the leaves, twigs and berries. A clear to pale yellow mobile liquid.

Fragrance
Woody, sharp, musty, slightly resinous

Cultivation/sustainability
WIldcrafted. No known sustainability issues

Principal Constituents
Terpenes: α-pinene, β-myrcene, limonene, sabinene, p-cymene, δ-cadinene, terpinen-4-ol, α-terpineol, β-phellandrene, β-caryophyllene, germacrene D

Actions:
Anti-inflammatory, antibiotic, antifungal, antimicrobial, antiseptic, astringent, balsamic, diuretic, expectorant,

Safety
No known cautions

Principal uses
Physical

» Arthritis
» Bronchitis,
» Diarrhea,
» Gum disease,
» Immune modulation,
» Lymphatic decongestant
» Ringworm
» Skin irritation
» Stomach bleeding
» Tumours

» Upper respiratory problems
» Urinary tract infections
» Wounds

Behavioural

» Aloof
» Disconnected
» Disturbed
» Hates confinement
» Self-harm
» Unsettling events

Think "Lentisk" for
Anytime there is dental issues, especially if the animal feels rundown or lethargic, or unsettled. Tumours and feelings of being stuck or entrapped.

LEMON

(Citrus Limon)

Element: Earth (Fire)

History and Character

A small citrus tree with glossy, evergreen leaves, small white flowers, and an abundance of yellow fruit. Native to Asia, it now grows wild in the southern Mediterranean and is widely cultivated. It is a very nutritious fruit and a great pick-me-up. Traditionally, it was used to protect against typhoid, malaria and scurvy. Physically, one of lemon's strongest actions is as an immune stimulant. It also has the ability to break down excessive build up of bone, for instance kidney stones. Traditionally horsemen used to strap half a lemon to a horse's leg as a cure of ringbone. Energetically, lemon is light, cleansing, refreshing, uplifting, sharpens focus and reduces confusion, helping to assimilate change and increase trust in oneself and others. Lemon is a simple soul with a wide range of uses and one of my personal favourites.

Synonyms

Limonum.

Cultivation/sustainability

Cultivated. Use organic

Extraction and Characteristics

Cold-pressed from the outer part of the fresh peel.

Fragrance

Sharp, sweet, clean with a bitter bottom note.

Principal Constituents

Terpenes: limonene, β-pinene, γ-terpinene, β-bisabolene, α-pinene, ρ-cymene
Aldehydes: geranial, neral

Actions

Anti-anaemic, antibacterial, anticoagulant, antifungal, anti-inflammatory, antisclerotic, antiseptic (air), antispasmodic (stomach), antiviral, astringent, calmative, carminative, digestive, diuretic, expectorant, immunostimulant, litholytic, pancreatic stimulant, phlebotonic, stomachic.

Safety

Non-toxic, may cause dermal irritation in some individuals, possible photo-toxicity, dilute below 2% on exposed skin.

Principal Uses

Physical:

- » Immune tonic
- » Kidney and liver congestion
- » Kidney stones
- » Bony growths

Behavioural:

- » Hyper alert animals
- » Issues of trust
- » Over-reactive animals

Think 'Lemon' for:

Hyperactive animals who tend to run when scared, especially if they are underweight or prone to illness or lack trust in themselves or their owner.

Bony growths.

LEMONGRASS

(Cymbopogon Citratus)

Element: Earth

History and Character

Lemongrass is a fast-growing tropical grass with long sharp leaves and a thick network of roots. Lemongrass has an invigorating, sharp, lemony scent, with a grassy, rooty undertone. Lemongrass is commonly used in soaps and cleaning products because of its fragrance and its antiseptic properties. It is also widely used in India, in Ayurvedic medicine to help bring down fevers and treat infectious illnesses; as a tea to calm stomach cramps; also as a pesticide and preservative for palm-leaf manuscripts. Lemongrass has also been used traditionally for arthritis and muscular pain. In 2006, researchers at the University of Ben Gurion in Israel found that lemongrass caused apoptosis (programmed cell death) in cancer cells. This oil is both stimulant and sedative, clearing the mind and grounding the body, relieving anxiety.

Synonyms

Andropogon citratus, West Indian lemongrass, A.Schoenathus.

Cultivation/sustainability

Cultivated. No known issues

Extraction and characteristics

Steam distilled from the fresh or partially dried grass. Pale yellow, to amber liquid.

Fragrance

Fresh, sharp, lemony, with earthy undertones.

Principal constituents

Aldehydes: citrate
Terpenes: myrcene, dipentene, methylheptenone
Alcohols: Linalol, geraniol, nerol, citronellol, farnesol

Actions

Analgesic, antidepressant, antimicrobial, antiseptic, antispasmodic, astringent, fungicidal, insecticidal, nervine, sedative (nervous system).

Safety

Generally held to be non-toxic, possibility of skin sensitisation, use at low dilutions.

Principal uses

Physical:
- » Viral infections
- » Nervous exhaustion
- » Soft tissue damage
- » Fungal infection
- » Lymphatic drainage
- » Insect repellent
- » Diarrhoea
- » Digestive upset
- » Sprains
- » Tendinitis
- » Neuralgia
- » Rheumatism
- » Tumours

Behavioural:
- » Depression
- » Confusion
- » Anxiety

Think 'Lemongrass' for:

In flea or fly spray, especially for animals who tend to be stiff.
Chronic problems of the digestive or musculo-skeletal system, especially if accompanied by depression or anxiety.

MANUKA

(Leptospermum Scoparium)

Element: Metal

History and Character

Manuka is a medium-sized shrub with small spiky leaves and pink flowers, which grows wild throughout New Zealand. The Maori used various parts of the plant for a wide range of complaints from head colds to fractures, and burns to dysentery. Captain Cook gave manuka the name of tea tree and wrote of it, "...the leaves were used by many of us as a tea which has a very agreeable bitter taste and flavour when they are fresh, but loses some of both when they are dried." Nowadays, it best known in manuka honey which is recommended by medical practitioners for its immune stimulant and bactericidal properties, especially for topical use on wounds and burns. The bactericidal properties of manuka are much higher in oil produced from the East Cape chemotype. Energetically, manuka is cleansing and nourishing and settles anxiety, very similar actions to tea tree oil but softer and more feminine.

Roza's Ringworm

Courtesy of Chrissie Slade, mGEOTA, proprietor of Gorgeous Guineas, Animal PsychAromaticist

Roza was a 4 year old rescued Guinea pig, who arrived in poor condition. She had been living with me for over a year and seemed healthy and happy.

Then one day, Roza's skin turned very red and irritated and she was diagnosed with ringworm. The infection was mostly on the right side of her body around the ear and surrounding skin, which felt very hot. Roza was also atypically grumpy.

In Traditional Chinese Medicine, Ringworm is associated with Damp Heat, so I chose oils to cool, calm her skin and disperse Damp: angelica root, for multiple problems, the "healing angel" and also anti-fungal. (1 drop in 10 ml), manuka — anti-inflammatory, antifungal, antibacterial, chamomile (German), anti-inflammatory, calming for itchy skin and stress manifesting in the body, also good for angry outbursts which she still has on the odd occasion.

Each essential oil was diluted individually 1 drop in 10ml calendula macerated oil, (anti-inflammatory, antifungal, emotionally comforting, cools and nourishes skin, clears Damp Heat and stimulates the lymphatic system). Within a couple of days there was a marked improvement in Roza's condition. Within 10 days Roza's skin was back to normal and in 14 days she had gone off all the oils. Roza spent up to 15 minutes with just one aroma at the beginning, and the first sessions took 30 minutes, gradually decreasing as she started going off the oils.

Synonyms
New Zealand Tea Tree.

Cultivation/sustainability
Wildcrafted. No known issues

Extraction and Characteristics
Steam distillation of the leaves and terminal branchlets of the East Cape chemotype of Leptospermum Scoparium. It is a pale amber liquid with a slightly oily texture.

Fragrance

Pungent, herbaceous aroma with a subtle spicy undertone.

Principal Constituents

Terpenes:α--pinene, cubebene, α-copaene, beta-selinene, α-selinene, cis calamanene, delta-cadinene,
cadina-1,4-diene,
Tri-ketones: flavesone, iso-leptospermone, leptospermone

Actions

Anti-allergenic, antibacterial (especially gram+ bacteria), antifungal, antihistamine, anti-inflammatory, antiseptic, insecticidal.

Safety

Generally held to be non-toxic, non-irritant, and non-sensitising.

Principal Uses

Physical:
  » Ringworm and other fungal infections
  » Skin eruptions
  » Ulcers and wounds, cuts and abrasions
  » Muscular aches and pain
  » Coughs, cold and flu
  » Bacterial infections and wound healing

Think 'Manuka' for:

Animals who are rundown especially if they have eruptive skin conditions or fungal infections or tend to be anxious. Staphylococcus or other gram-positive infections.

MARJORAM, SWEET

(Origanum majorana)

Element: Earth

History and Character

Sweet marjoram is a bushy perennial with small, hairy, dark green, oval leaves and tiny clustered white flowers. Native to the Mediterranean and North Africa it is not to be confused with Spanish marjoram (Thymus mastichina) or common marjoram (Origanum vulgare). A traditional cooking herb, its name comes from the Greek for "Joy in the mountain". The Greeks used the herb in fragrances and medicines and planted it on graves to bring spiritual peace to the departed, thus it is associated with grieving. Although marjoram's scent was said to be given by Aphrodite, goddess of love, it is considered an anaphrodisiac due to its ability to lower blood pressure. It is also deeply relaxing for muscles and psyche. Warming, nourishing and fortifying, this oil is comforting, like Grandmother's soup, good for those who feel that "nobody cares" and are needy for love. It can also help one come to terms with loss.

Synonyms
Majorana Hortensis.

Cultivation/sustainability
Wildcrafted. Vigourous healthy wild population

Extraction and Characteristics
Steam distillation from the dried flowering herb. It is a pale yellow liquid with a warm, herbaceous sweet fragrance.

Principal Constituents
Alcohols: terpinen-4-ol, cis-thujanol, trans-thujanol, α-terpineol, linalol

Terpenes: γ-terpinene, sabinene, myrcene, α-terpinene, terpinolene, paracymene, β-caryophyllene
Esters: geranyl acetate, terpenyl acetate

Actions
Analgesic, anaphrodisiac, antispasmodic, antiviral, bactericidal, calmative, digestive, diuretic, expectorant, hormone-like, hypotensive, neurotonic, respiratory tonic, stomachic, vaso-dilator.

Safety
Generally held to be non-toxic, non-irritant and non-sensitising.

Principal Uses
Physical:
 » Muscle cramps and stiffness
 » Strained muscles
 » Tachycardia
 » Palpitations
 » Hypertension
 » Colicky intestinal cramps
 » Excess sexual energy

Behavioural:
 » Loss of companion
 » Those who need constant emotional reassurance
 » Nervous exhaustion

Think 'Marjoram' for:
Animals that are prone to muscle problems and digestive upsets, especially if they are emotionally needy or have suffered a recent loss.

MELISSA/LEMON BALM

(Melissa officinalis)

Element: Fire (Wood)

History and character

This plant originated in the Mediterranean region but is now widely cultivated. It is a leafy perennial that grows to about 60 cm/2 ft and likes soil with a high iron content. Melissa means 'honey bee' in Greek, because bees love the nectar of this herb. The plant can be an invasive weed In the right conditions, so it is surprising that the essential oil is one of the most expensive on the market. This is because the small, white-pink flowers yield very little essential oil per kilo of plant matter. This is also why melissa is one of the most highly adulterated essential oils; often sold as a blend of lemongrass, citronella and synthetic chemicals.

Melissa has an illustrious past and is often mentioned by traditional medics, it was described by John Evelyn (1620 — 1706) as "sovereign for the brain, strengthening the memory, and powerfully chasing away melancholy." The essential oil is considered to be one of the most medicinally powerful in aromatherapy due to its anti-viral properties, especially for herpes; it is also an immune stimulant.

Melissa is tonic to the Heart, calming panic and hysteria, slowing the heartbeat and reducing blood pressure; it is relaxing without being sedative. In humans, it has been used successfully for ADHD, reducing hyperactivity and increasing focus. This oil strengthens the sense of self, and is particularly suited to the type of animal who is oversensitive, or easily traumatised by confrontation, becoming dependent on others for their sense of security; or those who have a suspicious outlook on life, with a sense of restlessness.

Synonyms
Balm, heart's delight.

Cultivation/sustainability
Cultivated

Extraction and characteristics
Steam distillation of flowering tops and leaves,the oil is a pale yellow liquid.

Principal constituents
Aldehydes: geranial, neral, citronellal
Terpenes: β-caryophyllene, α-copaene, germacrene-D
Alcohols: linalol
Ketones: methyl heptanone
Oxides: caryophyllene oxide
Esters: geranyl acetate

Actions
Analgesic, antidepressant, antihistaminic, anti-inflammatory, antiviral antispasmodic, bactericidal, carminative, hypotensive and sedative, vermifuge.

Safety
One of the most frequently adulterated essential oils. Sensitisation and dermal irritation are possible, use high dilutions. Do not use on individuals with hypersensitive, diseased or damaged skin. Do not use at more than 1% dilution. Do not give orally to any animal suffering from glaucoma.

Principal uses

Physical:
- » Immune stimulant
- » Allergies (skin and respiratory)
- » High blood pressure
- » Viral infection
- » Herpes
- » Sluggish digestion
- » Hormonal irregularity
- » Shock

Behavioural:
- » Anxiety
- » Hyperactivity
- » Nervousness
- » Confusion
- » Suspicious
- » Over-sensitive
- » Depression

Think 'Melissa' For:
Viral infections, especially herpes.

Nervous or hyperactive animals, especially if they are reactive to the moods of others or fall into depression or seem confused by life and have an under-active immune response, which might manifest as allergies.

MYRRH

(Commiphora Myrrha)

Element: Earth (Metal)

History and Character
Myrrh is a shrub or small tree with sturdy knotted branches, trifoliate aromatic leaves and small white flowers. The trunk exudes an oleoresin, which hardens into red-brown tears. The trees are native to Northeast Africa and Southwest Asia, especially the desert regions of the Red Sea; the name is derived from the Arabic for 'bitter'. Myrrh is the grand old statesman of essential oils, one of the first substances to be valued for its scent. The Ancient Egyptians valued it as a healing unguent, and burnt it to honour the dead; the Ancient Hebrews drank

it with wine to prepare themselves for religious ceremonies; Jesus was offered wine laced with myrrh on the cross to diminish his suffering. Myrrh is like a desert wind, drying out dampness and invigorating those who are slow, lethargic or run down. Myrrh frees thoughts that are caught in a pattern of restlessness, brings peace of mind, helps close wounds physically and emotionally and creates a quiet place inside to recover from loss or rejection.

Synonyms
Balsanodendrum Myrrha, Gum Myrrh, Common Myrrh, Hirabol Myrrh, Myrrha.

Cultivation/sustainability
Some cultivation, mostly wild-crafted. Check for sustainable harvest.

Extraction and Characteristics
Steam distillation from the crude resin or (more commonly) solvent extraction of the crude myrrh to make a resinoid. The resinoid is a thick brown viscous mass not pourable at room temperature. The essential oil is a pale amber, oily liquid that is very sticky.

Fragrance
Sweet/sharp balsamic smell, resinous and slightly camphoraceous.

Principal Constituents
Terpenes: furanoeudesma-1,3-diene, curzerene, lindestrene.
Ketones: curzerenone, 1,10 (15)-furanodien-6-one

Action
Antifungal, anti-inflammatory, antiseptic, antispasmodic, astringent, cardiac tonic, carminative, cicatrisant, expectorant, immunostimulant, sedative, stomachic, tonic, vulnerary.

Safety
Non-irritant, non-sensitising, possibly toxic in high concentrations. Avoid in pregnancy.

Principal Uses

Physical:
  » Fungal skin infections
  » Weeping wounds
  » Rain scald and mud-fever
  » Excess mucous

Behavioural:
  » Sadness
  » Weighed down by responsibility
  » Quiet anxiety
  » Over-concern for others
  » Grief, loss

Think "Myrrh" for:
Restless animals that worry about others especially if they are prone to damp, oozing skin conditions or excess mucous.
Those who are stoic about pain and past suffering, especially if they have breathing problems.

NEROLI

(Citrus aurantium)

Element: Fire

History and Character

The orange tree is a medium size flowering citrus with glossy green, heart-shaped leaves, a smooth grey bark and masses of fragrant white flowers. Three separate oils are made from the fruit, leaves and blossom of this generous tree. Neroli is made from the blossom. Native to China, orange trees are now widely cultivated in any Mediterranean climate. The oil is thought to be named after an Italian princess who introduced the fragrance to Italian society in the 17th century; it has long been favoured as a perfume and used for ladies of a nervous constitution. In the Middle East, orange blossom water is used for fainting fits and shock. It has a powerful ability to revive someone who is in a state of shock from emotional or physical trauma and is one of my 'must have' first aid oils.

One of the primary Heart oils, Neroli is highly uplifting and calming and steadies the nerves, (useful before vet visits, or other situations that provoke anxiety). Neroli heals sorrow held in the heart and eases the pain of loss or separation from a loved one.

Synonyms

Orange Blossom, Orange Flower, Citrus Bigaradia, Citrus Vulgaris.

Cultivation/sustainability

Cultivated. Use organic

Extraction and Characteristics

Steam distillation of the freshly picked flowers. It is a pale orange mobile liquid.

Fragrance

Sweet floral, bittersweet, cool, rich orangey.

Principal Constituents

Alcohols: linalol, trans-nerolidol, α-terpineol, geraniol, nerol
Terpenes: limonene, β-pinene
Esters: linalyl acetate, neryl acetate, geranyl acetate

Actions

Anticoagulant, antidepressant, antiseptic, antispasmodic, aphrodisiac, carminative, digestive, neurotonic, sedative and tonic.

Safety

Generally held to be non-toxic, non-irritant and non-sensitising.

Neroli for Felicity

Courtesy of Pauhla Whitaker, mGEOTA, Reiki master

Felicity, a yearling Alpaca had recently been weaned when she developed a habit of sucking on mouthfuls of hay all day, or nibbling her owners arm if possible. She refused to eat or engage with the rest of the herd, was generally unsettled and not thriving. To make matters worse, it was mid-winter and she started to drop weight dramatically. The vet suspected that the constant sucking without swallowing anything had caused her to develop ulcers and prescribed antacids, wormer and a general feed supplement, but he was happy for Fliss's owners to try using essential oils alongside the prescribed treatments.

When I visited, Fliss was friendly, well-socialised, not nervous, but very driven and slightly manic in her behaviour. I had it in mind to offer her neroli (Citrus aurantium) for loss of companion (in this case her mother), it also calms colicky pain and is calming and reassuring to the heart. But before I had a chance to of-fer it Fliss walked over to my oil box, stuck her nose into the tray and picked out a tiny 1 ml vial of neroli that was tucked right into the corner behind another bottle! I diluted the oil and offered it to her, she rubbed it into her muzzle and licked it from my hand enthusiastically several times.

Fliss showed interest in neroli for a month, but from the day I visited she stopped sucking hay and started to eat properly. When the spring grass started to grow, Felicity was given a new role as mentor to a field of juvenile alpacas, which fulfilled her emotionally and physically, and she's been happy and healthy ever since.

Principal Uses

Physical:

- » Shock
- » Nervous hysteria
- » Nervous colic
- » Chronic diarrhoea
- » Scars

Behavioural:

- » Separation anxiety
- » Sadness taken to the heart
- » Before stressful events (trips to the vet, shows etc.)

Think "Neroli" for:

Nervous, flighty animals with a history of stomach upsets

Depression, caused by outside circumstances (including illness) or a general feeling of sadness, especially if it was triggered by the loss of a companion.

NUTMEG

(Myristica Fragrans)

Element: Earth (Fire)

History and Character

Nutmeg is the seed of a fruit borne by a tall evergreen tree with a greyish brown trunk and dense foliage. The fruit is red or yellow and plum-shaped. The husk of the fruit is known as mace and is also used in cooking and as an essential oil. The tree is native to the Moluccas but is cultivated in Indonesia, Sri Lanka and the West Indies; however, the West Indian oil is considered inferior. Nutmeg has a long history of use as a culinary spice and has been used as a remedy for digestive and urinary disorders. It has also been used to strengthen and tone uterine muscles, especially during pregnancy. Nutmeg is a very warming oil physically and emotionally and helps us reconnect with our inner warmth, so is good for those who need a lot of emotional support. It is euphoric and must be used judiciously as long-term use or low dilutions can cause hallucinations and dizziness; however, high dilutions used correctly are very relaxing. This oil is very useful for animals who overreact to stimuli or cannot get enough love and tend to be hyperactive, especially used in combination with vetiver.

Synonyms

M. officinalis, M.aromata, Nux Moschata, Myristica.

Cultivation/sustainability

Cultivated or wildcrafted, no known issues

Extraction and Characteristics

Steam distillation from the worm-eaten seed (worms eat away the fixed oil and fats). The oil is a colourless to pale yellow mobile liquid.

Fragrance

Warm spicy/sharp fragrance with a slightly lemony top note settling to burnt wood.

Principal Constituents

Terpenes: sabinene, α-pinene, β-pinene, τ-terpinene, limonene, α-terpinene, ρ-cymene, terpinolene
Phenyl ethers: myristicin, elemicin, safrole
Alcohols: terpinen-4-ol, α-terpineol
Oxides: 1,8-cineole

Actions

Analgesic, anti-emetic, antirheumatic, antiseptic, antispasmodic, carminative, digestive, emmenagogic, psycho-active, reproductive stimulant, uterine tonic.

Safety

Generally non-toxic, non-irritant. Amounts larger than 5 ml can cause epileptic type fits, coma and death. Absolutely do not use in pregnancy except to facilitate delivery. Do not use with pethidine as it inhibits monoamine synthesis.

Principal Uses

Physical:
- » Rheumatism
- » Reproductive problems
- » Sluggish digestion
- » Tired muscles

Behavioural:
- » Emotionally needy
- » Hyperactivity
- » Excessive need to please others
- » Intense anxiety that leads to clumsiness

Think 'Nutmeg' for:

Animals that knock you over in their enthusiasm to greet you or try too hard to please, especially if they have a tendency towards digestive gas build up or tight muscles.
Animals who are depressed, having given up of receiving the attention they crave.

ORANGE, SWEET

(Citrus Sinensis)

Element: Wood

History and Character

Smaller than the bitter orange that produces neroli oil, the sweet orange tree is not so hardy and has softer, broader leaves. Native to China, it is now cultivated wherever there is a Mediterranean climate. The oil is expressed from the skin of the orange and is mainly produced in Israel, Brazil and North America. The dried peel of orange has been used in Chinese medicine for centuries, the sweet orange being thought to increase bronchial excretion; the tree is also a traditional sign of good luck and prosperity. In Europe the oil has been used for nervous disorders, heart problems, colic, asthma and melancholy.

Energetically this oil is very happy and positive, young and playful, and I use it a lot with youngsters as it is a gentle option for stomach upsets and nervousness that are not deep-rooted. Orange encourages a more playful outlook on life, helping to move built up stress and frustration. It is a good oil for the perfectionist and those who try too hard, encouraging a more easy-going attitude.

Synonyms
C.aurantium Var. Dulcis, C.aurantium Var. Sinensis, China orange, Portugal orange.

Cultivation/sustainability
Cultivated. Buy organic

Extraction and Characteristics
Cold-expression of the ripe outer peel. The oil is a pale, burnt orange, mobile liquid.

Fragrance
A sweet, fresh-fruity, warm odour.

Principal Constituents
Terpenes: limonene, β-myrcene, β-pinene
Alcohols: linalol
Ketones: carvone

Actions
Antispasmodic, calmative, carminative, cholagogic, digestive, hepatic, stomachic.

Safety
Generally held to be non-toxic, non-irritant and non-sensitising. It is important to use organic orange as regular cultivation uses high levels of pesticide can contaminate the oil.

Principal Uses

Physical:
- » Youngsters' tummy upsets
- » Mouth ulcers
- » Obesity
- » Constipation

Behavioural:
- » Nervous tension
- » Depression
- » Anxious to please
- » Insecure

Think 'Sweet Orange' for:
Young animals of a nervous disposition who feel stressed by learning to the point of explosion, especially if there is a history of stomach upsets or overeating.
A good 'helper' oil when a little lift is needed.

PATCHOULI

(Pogostomen Cablin)

Element: Earth

History And Character

A large (1m/3 ft), sturdy, perennial herb of the mint family, with small, white, pink-tinged flowers and large, fragrant leaves. The plant is native to tropical regions of Asia and is now extensively cultivated in Caribbean countries, but Indonesia is the main producer of essential oil, with China, Malaysia and India also contributing. Traditionally it has been used as a perfume, insect repellent, to treat colds, headaches, nausea and other digestive upsets, including halitosis. In Japan and Malaysia it is used as an antidote to snake bite. Energetically it is grounding, strengthening and warming, although the fragrance also cools and clarifies the mind. Patchouli relieves nervous tension and lightens the pressures of life; it is especially suitable for those who have an urge to escape from problems, or a tendency to cut themselves off from their body, which can manifest as frequent minor injuries or a high degree of stoicism.

Synonyms

P.commosum, P.hortensis, P.heyneasus and P.plectranthoides are all cultivated for their oils and all are known as patchouli oil.

Cultivation/sustainability

Cultivated

Extraction and Characteristics

Steam distilled from the young leaves and shoots. It is a viscous, golden brown to amber liquid.

Fragrance

Musky, sweet, earthy, rich, spicy.

Principal Constituents

Sesquiterpenes: α-bulnesene, α-humulene, α-patchoulene, β-caryophyllene, β-patchoulene, aromadendrene, elemene, guaiene, gurjunene, seychellene.
Sesquiterponols: patchoulol, selinenol
Oxides: caryophyllene oxide, bulnesene oxide

Actions

Antibacterial, anti-inflammatory, anti-infectious, antidepressant, anti-emetic, antifungal antiseptic, antitoxic, antiviral, aphrodisiac, astringent, cicatrisant, diuretic, febrifuge, insect repellent, nervine, phlebotonic, prophylactic, stomachic.

Safety
Non-toxic, non-irritant

Principal Uses

Physical:

- » Damaged skin
- » Diarrhoea
- » Fungal skin infections
- » Immune imbalance
- » Insect and snake bites
- » Insect repellent
- » Nervous exhaustion
- » Sexual dysfunction
- » Sore back
- » Strained muscles
- » Viral infections

Behavioural:

- » Depression
- » Anxiety
- » Nervous tension
- » Insecurity that needs physical reassurance
- » Emotional collapse
- » Mental confusion

Think 'patchouli' for:
Animals who tend to take too much responsibility on themselves and become emotionally exhausted or physically uncomfortable and grumpy
Fungal infections, especially in summer

PEPPERMINT

(Mentha Piperita)

Element: Earth (Wood and Metal)

History and Character
A perennial herb up to 1 m/3 ft high with strong underground runners, green stems and leaves. There is also a black peppermint which has dark green serrated leaves and purplish stems. There are records of peppermint being used in Ancient Egypt, and the Romans and Greeks used it to perfume their beds, and in wine. Pliny said, "The very smell of it recovers and refreshes the spirit". It is one essential oil that is officially classified as a medicine for digestive problems, such as colitis and irritable bowel syndrome. Peppermint has a unique hot/cold effect when applied to the skin, so can be used along with hot/cold treatment for lameness in horses. Energetically, peppermint is invigorating and awakening, bringing things into focus mentally and emotionally. It helps animals to be clear about their boundaries so it is easy to take in and give out without defensiveness and with discrimination.

Synonyms
Brandy Mint, Balm Mint.

Cultivation/sustainability
Cultivated

Extraction and Characteristics
Steam distillation from the flowering herb. It is a pale yellow to green mobile liquid.

Fragrance
Cool, fresh, minty, pungent and green, slightly sweet.

Principal Constituents
Alcohols: menthol, neomenthol, viridiflorol
Ketones: menthone, iso-menthone, neomenthone, piperitone
Esters: menthyl acetate
Oxides: 1,8-cineole
Others: Menthofuran

Actions
Analgesic, antibacterial, anti-inflammatory, anti-lactogenic, anti-migraine, antiseptic, antispasmodic, antiviral, carminative, decongestant, digestive, expectorant, hepatic, hormone-like (ovarian stimulant), hypertensor, insect repellent, mucolytic, neurotonic, reproductive stimulant (impotence), uterotonic.

Safety
Generally held to be non-toxic. Do not use with children. Use in high dilutions on skin. Do not use on broken skin. Do not use in conjunction with homeopathy.

Principal Uses
Physical:
  » As a local anaesthetic
  » Tendon injury
  » To reduce swelling for aches, pains and strains
  » Digestive upsets
  » Colic
  » Colitis
  » Nerve damage
  » Asthma and bronchitis
  » Congested sinuses
  » Irritable bowel syndrome

Behavioural:
  » Animals who are bullied or bully others
  » Animals who are sensitive about their personal space
  » Defensive aggression
  » Lack of concentration

Think 'Peppermint' for:
Animals who display nervous aggression or over-defensiveness of their personal space, especially if they lack focus and suffer from digestive problems or asthma.
Tendon damage.

PLAI

(Zingiber cassumunar)

Element: Water (Earth)

History and Character

Approximately 60 cms/2 ft in height, plai has grass like lancelet leaves which die down each year. The flower stalk bearing white or yellow flowers grows directly from the root. The tuberous root is thick and white inside with a wonderful characteristic ginger scent. Plai is native to Thailand where it has been used for medicinal purposes for centuries, particularly to combat joint and muscle problems. It is closely related to Zingiber officinalis but does not possess the heat typical of 'common' ginger. Plai has a unique cooling action on inflamed areas, be they joints and muscles, or kidneys and lungs. It is said that undiluted plai can ease pain in inflamed joints for upwards of 18 hours. Plai has also been used to counter irritable bowel syndrome and for asthma. Plai from central Thailand has a significant percentage of dimethoxyphenyl butadiene, known for its analgesic effects. Plai is energetically cooling, allowing animals who are wound up or hot-tempered to feel more grounded and trusting.

Synonyms

Zingiber Purpureum Roscoe, Thai ginger.

Cultivation/sustainability

Cultivated.

Extraction and characteristics

Steam distilled from the fresh or dried root.

Fragrance

Cool, green, pungent, with a hint of earth.

Principal constituents

Monoterpenes: α-phellandrene, α-pinene, α-terpinene, α-thuyene, β-myrcene, β-phellandrene, β-pinene, γ-terpinene, d-limonene, para-cymene, sabinene, terpinolene
Sesquiterpenes: β-sesquiphellandrene, dimethoxyphenyl butadiene
Monoterpenols:α-terpineol, cis-thuyanol, terpinen-4-ol, trans-thuyanol

Actions

Analgesic, anti-neuralgic, anti-inflammatory, antiseptic, antispasmodic, antitoxic, antiviral, carminative, digestive, diuretic, febrifuge, laxative, rubefacient, stimulant, tonic and vermifuge.

Safety
No known safety issues.

Principal uses

Physical:
- » Asthma
- » Catarrh
- » Digestive upset
- » Fevers
- » Inflammation of joints and muscles
- » Influenza
- » Respiratory problems
- » Soft tissue damage, sprains and strains

Behavioural:
- » Bad tempered
- » Agitated
- » Impatient
- » Confused

Think "Plai" for:
For any musculo-skeletal pain or injury, especially if the animal is bad-tempered or worn down by its injury, has an occasional dry cough, or digestion is disturbed.

RAVENSARA

(Ravensara Aromatica)

Element: Metal

History and Character
A smallish tree with strongly aromatic bark and dark, smooth evergreen leaves, native to Madagascar. The name means "aromatic leaf", traditionally its flowers and seeds have been used as a spice and a universal remedy for physical and mental disorders. The leaves are used for the preparation of ointments and cough mixtures, extracts of the bark and leaves are used for indigestion. Ravensara is a strong immune-stimulant with particular affinity to the respiratory system. Iis said to be a good oil to use in conjunction with other oils as it supports and strengthens them. Energetically it is very sharp and penetrative giving strength and clarity to all systems so you can face the world with relaxed awareness and a strong sense of your own boundaries.

Synonyms
Ravensara Aromatica Gmelin, Evodia Ravensara Gaertn., Evodia Aromatica Poir., Agathophyllum Aromaticum Willd., Ravensara Anisata Danguy (this is in fact a different plant but often confused).

Cultivation/sustainability
Wildcrafted. No known issues

Extraction and Characteristics
Steam distillation from the leaves, the oil is a colourless liquid.

Fragrance
Spicy, sharp, camphoraceous, slightly liquorice tinted.

Principal Constituents
Terpenes: α-pinene, β-pinene, sabinene, β-caryophellene
Alcohols: α-terpineol, terpinen-4-ol
Esters: terpenyl acetate
Oxides: 1,8-cineole

Actions
Antibacterial, anti-inflammatory, antiseptic, antiviral, detoxicant, expectorant, neurotonic.

Safety
No contraindications known for Ravensara aromatica, however Ravensara anisata derived from the bark of the same tree, has substantial estragole and trans-anethole and is not to be used internally or externally in aromatherapy.

Principal Uses

Physical:
- » Viral infections
- » Herpes
- » Colds
- » Respiratory infection
- » Sinus infection
- » General immune stimulant
- » Neuromuscular problems

Think 'Ravensara' for:
Compromised immune systems, especially for those who feel unable to cope with life and new experiences in particular.

RHODODENDRON

(Rhododendron anthopogon)

Element: Fire (Metal)

History and Character
Rhododendron essential oil is distilled from the dwarf rhododendron, Rhododendron anthopogon. This small evergreen shrub is part of the Ericaceae family, members of which generally thrive in acidic soil and infertile, moist, growing conditions. Although there are

hundreds of varieties of Rhododendrons, this is the only variety that is non-toxic and the only one that can be distilled.

Anthopogon is considered to be one of the smallest plants in the Rhododendron genus growing no more than 1 metre high (2-3 feet). It thrives in the high altitudes of the Himalayan mountain range, across Nepal, Pakistan, northern India, Bhutan and SE Tibet. The plant is mainly harvested in Nepal. Its leathery leaves are the most aromatic part of the plant.

Called "Sunpati" in its native Nepal, it is a national symbol and revered for its medicinal use. The flowers and leaves are often used in native medicine for digestive and respiratory disorders. More specifically, it is thought to promote digestive fire and combat wet catarrh. Mountain climbers have used the tea to help with their endurance and it is known to relax tight muscles, being analgesic and anti-inflammatory. The stems and leaves of the sub-species R. anthopogon hypenanthum are used in Tibetan herbalism. They have a sweet, bitter and astringent taste and are used to treat lack of appetite, coughing and various skin disorders. In Nepal, the leaves are boiled and the vapour inhaled to treat coughs and colds.

The Department of Pharmaceutical Sciences, University of Padova, Italy documented strong inhibitory effect of the oil on a wide range of bacteria.

It is historically connected with meditation as it is used in incense by Buddhist monks. Energetically it is very calming, relaxing the mind, giving the uplifting feeling of being on the top of a hill in open air. It is helpful for those who get tightly wound and run on adrenalin, helping them to get grounded, stop for a minute, and take a wider view.

This oil provides support to a healthy respiratory system, is a general tonic, and strongly supports adrenal and liver function.

Synonyms
Dwarf rhododendron

Cultivation/sustainability
Wild harvested. Possibility of over-harvesting, check your supplier's policy to make sure harvesting is monitored for sustainability

Extraction
Steam distilled from leaves and flowers. Clear mobile liquid.

Fragrance
Balsamic, floral, slightly camphoraceous, sweet, exotic

Principal Constituents
Monoterpenes: α-pinene, β-pinene, limonene, (Z)-β-ocimene, γ-terpinene, β-myrcene, (E)-β-ocimene,δ-cadinene, β-caryophyllene, α-muurolene, γ-cadinene, γ-muurolene, β-selinene, α-selinene

Oxide: 1,8 cineole
Alcohols: linalool, citronellol, fenchol, borneol, geraniol, nerol

Actions
Analgesic, Anti-anxiety, Anti-bacterial, Anti-depressant, Anti-fungal, Anti-inflammatory, Anti-oxidant, Anti-spasmodic, Decongestant, Immuno-stimulant

Safety
Considered Non-toxic, non-irritant, non-sensitizing

Principal uses

Physical
- » Tight muscles
- » Coughs and colds
- » Bronchitis
- » Allergic respiratory distress
- » Adrenal exhaustion
- » Diarrhoea
- » Excess mucous

Behavioural
- » Anxiety
- » Extreme startle response
- » Nervous tension
- » Hyperactive
- » Restlessness

Think 'Rhododendron ' for
Animals who find it hard to relax, especially if they have excess mucous or digestive upsets.

ROSALINA

(Melaleuca Ericifolia)

Element: Metal

History and Character
Native to Australia, Rosalina is a tall, shrub, 6-9 m/20-30 ft high with a bushy top and greyish papery bark, with soft, alternate, smooth and narrow linear leaves. Similar to Melaleuca alternifolia, rosalina produces new top growth readily after severe cutting. It grows in low-lying swamps, along creeks and behind sand dunes in Australia. It is similar to tea tree in its actions but because of its high linalol content is very gentle on the skin. It is a gentle 'yin' oil, very cooling and relaxing and tender.

Synonyms
Australian Rosalina, Lavender Tea Tree, Swamp Paperbark.

Cultivation/sustainability
Mostly wildcrafted. No known issues

Extraction and Characteristics
Steam distillation from leaves and small twigs.

Fragrance
Sharp, camphoraceous, slightly sweet herbaceous.

Principal Constituents
Alcohols: linalol.
Oxides: 1,8 cineole.
Terpenes: α-pinene, aromadendrene.

Actions
Antibacterial, anti-inflammatory, antiseptic, detoxicant, expectorant, febrifuge, sedative.

Safety
Generally held to be non-toxic, non-irritant and non-sensitising.

Principal Uses

Physical:
- » Wounds
- » Boils
- » Respiratory infections
- » Fevers
- » Bladder infections

Think 'Rosalina' for:
Infected wounds or respiratory conditions, especially if the immune system is low due to stress.

ROSE

(Rosa Damascena)

Element: Fire

History and Character
Rose oil comes from the Damask Rose, a bush rose up to 2 m/6 ft high with highly fragrant, pink, 36-petalled blooms. Originally a product of the orient, roses are now cherished all over the world, however the best oil is produced in Bulgaria and some parts of Turkey. 'The queen of flowers', dedicated to Aphrodite, rose is one of the most yin essential oils and its cooling properties are second to none. It is also cathartic, helping to release energy blocked because of emotional wounds, which often manifests as resentfulness and an attitude of, "I will reject you before you can reject me". It balances the physical and emotional body and allows the heart to be receptive, restoring trust in oneself and others. It also has a powerful effect on the hormonal system.

Synonyms
Summer Damask Rose, Bulgarian Rose, Turkish Rose, Rose Otto, Attar of Roses.

Cultivation/sustainability
Cultivated. Choose organic

Extraction and Characteristics
Steam distillation of the fresh petals. The oil is a yellow to pale green colour.

Rose for self-love

I was asked to help a horse that belonged to a young girl suffering from anorexia. The horse had become very withdrawn and self-protective and tried to bite anyone coming into her stall. When I met her, her blanket had not been removed in days, as no-one dared try. The mare was standing in the far corner of a large loose-box, when I put my hand on the latch of the door she flattened her ears at me threateningly. I removed the lid from the bottle of undiluted rose and held it over the door without looking at the mare. Rose helps to release resentful anger turned in on oneself to cause self harm.

I stood there in a quiet, unthreatening manner as the horse gently inched her way towards the bottle. After about five minutes I felt her breathe gently on my hand, and glancing at her I could see she was going into a trance. Then I withdrew the bottle, diluted a drop of the rose in 5 ml of sunflower oil and put it on my hand.

Slowly I opened the door and reached my hand towards the mare. She looked at me, sniffed my hand and licked a little. I offered to touch her neck with the rose, she flinched slightly but did not object. Once I got my hand on her she relaxed completely and allowed me to rub her chest, I then removed her blanket and continued to rub her all over her body, letting her smell the rose again whenever she asked. Other oils she consequently chose were angelica root and vanilla. This was the beginning of a healing journey for both horse and girl.

Fragrance
Rich, sweet, floral, slightly astringent, with a subtly spicy edge.

Principal Constituents
Alcohols: citronellol, geraniol, nerol, phenyl ethanol, linalol, farnesol
Terpenes: stearoptene
Hyrdocarbons: nonadecane
Esters: geranyl acetate, neryl acetate
Phenyl ethers: methyl eugenol

Actions

Antibacterial, antidepressant, anti-inflammatory, antiseptic, astringent, cicatrizant, general tonic, neurotonic, sexual tonic, styptic.

Safety

Generally held to be non-toxic, non-irritant and non-sensitising.

Principal Uses

Physical:
> » Irregular hormonal cycle
> » Inability to conceive
> » Liver deficiency

Behavioural:
> » Past abuse

> » Nervous restlessness
> » Debility
> » Resentful anger
> » Moody mares
> » Self harm/mutilation

Think 'Rose' for:

Those who turn anger on themselves, especially females who are moody or irritable when in season, or there is a history of past abuse, or males who are resentful about past treatment.

ROSEMARY

(Rosmarinus Officinalis)

Element: Fire (Earth)

History and Character

A strongly aromatic evergreen shrub up to 2 m/6 ft high, it is native to the Mediterranean but widely cultivated as a culinary herb. Rosemary has an affinity to the head, stimulating the brain and encouraging hair growth. The old saying "Rosemary for remembrance" derives from its ability to enhance concentration and brain activity, also because it was burnt at the funerals of the Greeks and Romans. In the Middle Ages in France, rosemary was burnt to disinfect the air in hospitals. It was also used as a general panacea as it was reputed to strengthen the body and the brain. Energetically, rosemary is a very stimulating herb while being strongly earthed and with a 'can do' attitude. It bolsters self-confidence and lends courage to those who doubt their own abilities.

Synonyms

Compass Plant, Incesier.

Cultivation/sustainability

Cultivated or wildcrafted. No issues

Extraction and Characteristics
Steam distillation of the fresh flowering tops and leaves. The oil is a colourless to pale yellow liquid.

Fragrance
Green-herbaceous, camphoraceous, slightly sweet and warm.

Principal Constituents
(Rosemary has a variety of chemotypes which will affect make-up)
Oxides: 1,8 cineole
Ketones: verbenone, camphor
Terpenes: α-pinene, camphene, β-pinene, myrcene, limonene, β-caryophyllene
Alcohols: borneol, α-terpineol, linalol

Actions
Analgesic, antibacterial, antifungal, anti-inflammatory, antiseptic, antispasmodic, antitussive, antiviral, cardiotonic, carminative, choleretic, cicatrizant, detoxicant, digestive, diuretic, emmenagogue, enuresis, hyperglycaemic, hypertensor, hypotensive, litholytic, lowers cholesterol, mucolytic, neuromuscular, neurotonic, sexual tonic, stimulant (adrenal cortex), venous decongestant.

Safety
Generally held to be non-toxic, non-irritant and non-sensitising. Use in high dilutions. There are conflicting opinions as to its safety in pregnancy and epilepsy, I suggest not to use it in these cases.

Principal Uses

Physical:
- » Sluggish circulation
- » Navicular disease
- » Overworked muscles
- » Respiratory congestion
- » Hair loss or patchy coats
- » Tight muscles

Behavioural:
- » Nervous animals
- » Lack of confidence
- » Disconnected emotionally or mentally

Think 'Rosemary' for:
Nervous animals with patchy coats, who lack confidence in their abilities which often manifests as an inability to concentrate.
Horses on box rest to stimulate their minds and their circulation.

SEAWEED, BLADDERWRACK

(Fucus vesiculosus)

Element: Water

History and Character

Bladderwrack grows in cold coastal waters in the Atlantic Ocean and is also cultivated in farms for a contaminant-free product. Thick, pale stems anchor long, dark rubbery fronds (up to 60m/200 ft) to the ocean floor. The seaweed acts as a filter, absorbing toxins and cleaning debris from the ocean, the essential oil/absolute also work in this way drawing toxins out of the body. One of the signatures of this plant is its constant movement, which is why we use it for conditions that don't move, chronic problems, severe lameness, or whenever body or energy is blocked. Seaweed is also a source of vital trace minerals, a source of revitalisation. It has a cooling, soothing and nourishing energy, giving relief wherever things are blocked, overheated, or seem unbearable.

Synonyms

Kelp.

Cultivation/sustainability

Wild crafted.

Extraction and Characteristics

Alcohol distillation of a solvent-extracted concrete. It is highly viscous, dark green and sticky.

Fragrance

A distinctive 'seashore' odour; salty, green and fresh with a musty undertone.

Principal Constituents

Esters: ethyl oleate, ethyl palmitate, ethyl myristate, ethyl linolate
Hydrocarbons: pentadecane

Actions

Alterative, antacid, anti-allergenic, anti-arthritic/rheumatic, antibacterial, anticandida, anticoagulant, anti-inflammatory, antioxidant, antisclerotic, antitoxin, antiviral, aperient, detoxicant, diuretic, hypotensive.

Safety

Generally held to be non-toxic, non-irritant and non-sensitising. Use with caution with vulnerable animals. Contraindicated in hyperthyroidism. Use in moderation if on a detox programme, to avoid discomfort.

Seaweed gets Emmie Moving

Courtesy of Mary Lindo VN, mGEOTA

Emmie was an 18- year-old domestic longhair tabby cat who had been with her owner from the age of eight weeks. Emmie had several health problems: a slight heart murmur; her thyroid gland had been removed because it was over-active; and blood tests had shown mild renal failure for the last three years. Emmie's person's main focus was that Emmie's quality of life should be as good as possible for the time she had left. The focus of her essential oil treatment was her arthritic hips.

Emmie needed just one oil, seaweed. Seaweed stimulates the circulation of blood, draws toxins out of cells and improves osmotic change and waste elimination. It is anti-inflammatory, aids lack of movement, dissipates swelling, and immune stimulant. It is a nourishing oil, good for kidney problems and contains an abundance of vitamins and minerals. Seaweed is also very supportive of the body's endocrine functions.

The seaweed absolute was diluted 1 drop in 10 ml of passionflower macerated oil. The dilution was offered to Emmie twice daily for 11 days. She inhaled it, frequently going into a trance for a few minutes. She never wanted to lick it. During this time her appetite improved and she became much less picky about what she ate, her coat became silky and shiny, her mobility improved, her back legs were straighter and she could jump onto chairs easily.

Emmie's person continued to offer her the oil regularly, but Emmie only showed occasional interest. Six months later Emmie was quietly put to sleep when her kidney disease became too bad. Emmie's person was very happy with her beloved cat's quality of life over the last summer, and that she had been able to help her in such a simple and non-invasive way.

Principal Uses

Physical
- » Chronic illnesses that are static
- » Degenerative disease
- » Immune stimulant
- » Laminitis
- » Navicular disease
- » Arthritis
- » Poisoning
- » Cushing's disease
- » Metabolic syndrome
- » Swellings and inflammations
- » Thyroid problems

Behavioural
- » When fear has become frozen
- » Extreme lack of self confidence
- » Depression
- » Lack of motivation

Think 'Seaweed' for:

Animals who are run-down or have any chronic condition especially if any of the symptoms suggest 'lack of movement'.

Lumps, and soft bumps, especially if animal is withdrawn, lethargic or has weight problems.

SPEARMINT

(Mentha Spicata)

Element: Earth

History and Character

A creeping perennial herb with bright green leaves and spires of white or pale pink flowers, native to Europe but widely cultivated and valued as a food flavouring. It is similar to peppermint in its actions but softer, gentler and more nurturing which makes it very suitable for use with youngsters and oldsters. It soothes away problems rather than cutting through them and is excellent for dull insistent pain of any sort.

Synonyms

M. Viridis, M. Crispa. Spire Mint, Green Mint, Lamb Mint.

Cultivation/sustainability

Cultivated

Extraction and Characteristics

Steam distillation from the flowering tops. The oil is a pale yellow to green liquid.

Fragrance

Warm, sweet herbaceous, spicy green fragrance.

Principal Constituents

Ketones: carvone, dihydrocarvone
Terpenes: limonene, pinene, β-myrcene
Oxides: 1,8 cineole

Actions:

Anaesthetic (local), antiseptic, antispasmodic, astringent, carminative, decongestant, digestive, diuretic, expectorant, febrifuge, hepatic, neurotonic, stimulant, stomachic, tonic.

Safety

Generally held to be non-toxic, non-irritant and non-sensitising.

Principal Uses

Physical:

- » Digestive disorders
- » Flatulence and nausea
- » To clear respiratory mucous
- » Allergy related respiratory problems
- » Circulatory problems, muscle spasms and cramps
- » Young animals
- » Anaesthetic

Think 'Spearmint' for:

A young animal with digestive or respiratory problems especially if they have problems with hierarchy, or older animals with persistent dull pain internally or externally.

BLUE TANSY

(Tanacetum anuum)

Element: Metal (Fire)

History and Character

Blue tansy is is a member of the asteraceae family native to the Mediterranean. It is an annual plant that grows to 40 centimetres in height, with small, yellow button heads that bloom from August to October. It is often confused with perennial common tansy, or Tanacetum vulgare, but they have a quite different chemical profile and essential oil of common tansy is toxic. There is no historically distinct references to the use of the annual tansy, but as an essential oil it is a safe and gentle anti-inflammatory, like all the 'blue' oils high in chamazulene. Personally it is a recent addition to my kit. I started using it when it became impossible to source a good Great Mugwort. I was reluctant to use it because of sustainability issues, but these seem to be somewhat alleviated by an increase in cultivation of the plant, rather than indiscrimnate wild-harvesting. I use the oil mostly for its anti-histamine effect, especially over-reactivity to fly/flea bites. It also works well for seasonal allergies, sinusitis and wheezing. Energetically it appears to settle the nerves and calm restlesss behaviour.

Synonyms

Annual tansy, Moroccan chamomile, blue chamomile

Cultivation/sustainability

Some cultivation. Has been over-harvested in the wild, so prefere cultivated or check supply chain carefully.

Extraction

Steam distilled from flowering tips. The whole is a deep blue, turning slightly green with age.

Fragrance
Green herbaceous, slightly camphoraceous, with a sweet, fruity edge.

Principal Constituents
Terpenes: sabinene, chamazulene, camphor, p-cymene, β-myrcene,, 1,8 cineole, 3,6-Dihydrochamazulene,

Actions
Analgesic, antihistaminic, anti-inflammatory, anti-allergenic, antibacterial, antifungal, antimicrobial, antispasmodic, antiviral, diaphoretic, expectorant, febrifuge, nervine, sedative, tonic.

Safety
Tisserand and Young caution that a drug interaction may occur when using drugs metabolized by CYP2D6. The essential oil is contra-indicated for use with women who have an endocrine imbalance and in pregnancy. In addition, do not use in dilution above 5%.

Principal uses

Physical
  » Allergic reaction in skin or lungs
  » Fungal skin infections
  » Hot spots
  » Excessive itching

Behavioural
  » Restless irritability

Think 'Tansy' for
Any hot itchy condition, especially if the animal is nervous or flighty or disturbed by minor irritations.
Allergies

TEA TREE

(Melaleuca Alternifolia)

Element: Metal

History and Character
Tea tree is a small tree with needle-like leaves and small yellow or purplish flowers. Native to Australia, the Aboriginal people used its leaves in a tea for fevers, colds, and headaches. It has been extensively researched in recent years and found to be a powerful immunostimulant and active against bacteria, fungi and viruses. Energetically, it is tremendously cleansing, fortifying the lungs and giving confidence. It is useful for those who feel victimised or unable to cope with worldly matters.

Synonyms
Ti-tree, Narrow-leaved Paperbark Tree, Ti-trol, Melasol.

Cultivation/sustainability
Mostly cultivated.

Extraction and Characteristics
Steam distillation of the leaves and twigs. A clear mobile liquid.

Fragrance
A strongly camphoraceous, medicinal odour.

Principal Constituents
Alcohols: terpinen-4-ol, α-terpineol, globulol, viridiflorol
Terpenes: γ-terpinene, α-terpinene, para-cymene, terpinolene, α-pinene, limonene, δ-cadinene, aromadendrene, viridiflorene
Oxides: 1,8 cineole

Actions
Antibacterial, antifungal, antiseptic, antiparasitic, antiviral, expectorant, febrifuge, immunostimulant.

Safety
Generally held to be non-toxic, non-irritant and non-sensitising. Levels of para-cymene rise in old or improperly stored tea tree making skin reaction more likely. Tea tree has caused temporary paralysis in dogs when used undiluted. Never use tea tree with cats.

Principal Uses

Physical
- » Wound disinfectant
- » Skin infections
- » Boils
- » Abscesses
- » Immune stimulant
- » Fever
- » Strangles

Think 'Tea tree' for:
First aid, cleaning wounds and abscesses or infected wounds, or thrush in horses feet.

THYME

(Thymus Vulgaris)

Element: Metal (Water)

History and Character

Thyme is a small, evergreen shrub with tiny fragrant leaves and woody stems. Thyme is native to the hot, rocky slopes of the Mediterranean but is cultivated throughout the world. It was used by the Egyptians for embalming and by the Greeks to clean the air of infection because of its anti-bacterial nature. It has been widely used as a cooking herb, especially to preserve meat, testament to its antibacterial properties. In Western herbal lore, thyme has been used for respiratory infections and digestive problems. Energetically, thyme is very warm and dry, especially the thymol chemotype, inspiring yang energy to flow smoothly. Thyme infuses the Kidney meridian with warmth, stimulating us at an essential level to overcome fear. This is supported by thyme's stimulant action on the lungs, which encourages deep, regular breathing. I call it the Brave oil.

Synonyms

Common Thyme, Garden Thyme.

Cultivation/sustainability

Cultivated or wild-crafted. No known issues

Extraction and Characteristics

The essential oil is obtained by water or steam distillation from the fresh or partially dried leaves and flowering tops. 'Red thyme' oil is obtained from the first distillation and 'white' thyme oil is produced by further distillation. The oil is a clear mobile liquid and the colour can be anywhere from rusty red to pale yellow depending on the chemotype.

Fragrance

Warm, herbaceous, sweet, medicinal.

Principal Constituents

There are two main chemotypes of thyme sold today, these are thymol, which is strongly disinfectant and harsh on the skin and linalol, less disinfectant but much more gentle on the skin and psyche.

Actions

Anthelmintic, antiseptic, antispasmodic, antitoxic, carminative, diuretic, expectorant, hypertensive, rubefacient, stimulant and vermifuge.

Safety

Due to the high content of the phenols carvacrol and thymol, certain chemotypes can irritate mucous membranes, cause dermal irritation and may cause sensitisation in susceptible animals. The essential oil should be used in low concentrations. It is contraindicated with high blood pressure. The alcohol-rich chemotypes are much safer to use.

Principal Uses

Physical:
- » Respiratory problems, excess mucous
- » Digestive disease and diarrhoea
- » Circulatory stagnation
- » Bacterial infections
- » Thrush

Behavioural:
- » Lethargy
- » Despondency
- » Animals who lack courage

Think 'Thyme' for:

Fearful animals who feel overwhelmed by responsibility.
Defensive aggression, especially if there is a tendency to produce excess mucous or diarrhoea.
Aggressive bacterial infection.

VALERIAN ROOT

(Valeriana Officinalis)

Element: Water

History and Character

A perennial herb growing to 1.5 metres/5 ft tall, with a hollow stem, deeply dissected leaves and masses of purple/pink flowers. The roots are short and thick and mostly show above ground. There are many species of valerian around the world and it has been used for conditions such as nervous tension, backache, intestinal colic; its mediaeval name was All Heal. It is a painkiller and a powerful sedative. Valerian is one of the most stabilising of essential oils, and can be used when the mind is overcome by emotion, leading to panic, hysteria or frozen fear. It slows the world down so the situation does not seem to be so overwhelming. I often use it when all the stress circuits are 'blown', resulting in extremes of fearful or aggressive behaviour.

Synonyms

Common Valerian, Garden Heliotrope

Cultivation/sustainability

Mostly wild-crafted. No sustainability issues

Valerian Calms Berry's Barking

Courtesy of Caroline Thomas, APA graduate, Reiki healer, Bach flower practitioner.

Berry, a three-year-old border collie, was frightened of cars, lying down frozen when they passed; hot air balloons and fireworks; men, especially strangers. Berry barks non-stop at anything or anyone. In the living room she will not settle, constantly running in circles, jumping on anything or everything. Her people did not have many visitors because of this.

Berry was purchased at 15 weeks old, a time in a dog's life that new things are particularly scary, so being introduced to new things at this time can create a nervous dog. Also Berry is fed a commercial dried food and does not eat it at once when it is put down but will save her morning feed till late afternoon. I suggested they change to a more natural diet.

The essential oils Berry needed were frankincense, for fear of known things, and valerian, for hyper-reactive fear. The essential oils were diluted in a base of hypericum macerated oil 2 drops in 5 ml and 4 drops in 5 ml respectively.

Berry was keenly interested in both oils for six days, then she started to be less interested in the frankincense and lost interest completely by day nine. She carried on taking the valerian, licking a few drops twice a day for a further five days, when she lost interest completely.

By day four, when workmen came into the house Berry stayed quiet if a little nervous. Her person said that by the time Berry lost interest in the oils her behaviour had improved by 85%, . Because Berry is calmer, the whole house now has a calm energy.

Extraction and Characteristics

The oil is obtained by steam distillation of the rhizomes and root of the plant. They are usually picked in the second year after the leaves have dried off. It is a viscous light brown liquid.

Fragrance

Sweet, licorice-like, musty, warm. The fragrance can be overpowering.

Principal Constituents

Terpenes: camphene, α-pinene, β-pinene, limonene, α-fenchene
Esters: bornyl acetàte, myrtenyl acetate

Actions

Anodyne, antispasmodic, carminative, diuretic, hypotensive, regulator, sedative, stomachic.

Safety
Non-toxic and non-irritant however some sensitisation has been reported in humans. It has a strongly sedating effect use in moderation and well diluted.

Principal Uses

Physical:
- » Shock
- » Sedation

Behavioural:
- » Chronic fear

- » Fear of known things
- » Hysteria
- » Panic
- » Pathological insecurity

Think 'Valerian' for:
Animals who become hysterical when fearful, especially of known things or if their adrenal system has been overloaded.

VANILLA

(Vanilla planifolia)

Element: Earth

History and Character
A herbaceous vine that climbs to 25 metres/80 ft high, bearing large white trumpet-shaped flowers. The oil is extracted from the beans, which grow inside long, brown pods. It is native to Central America and Mexico and is a key ingredient of chocolate. Vanilla is energetically sweet, rich and nourishing and soothes and sweetens the sharpest of moods.

Synonyms
Mexican Vanilla, Bourbon Vanilla.

Cultivation/sustainability
Cultivated. No known issues. Buy fairtrade to make sure the farmers who grow it earn enough.

Extraction and Characteristics
A resinoid by solvent extraction from the cured vanilla beans.

Principal Constituents
Vanillin, hydroxybenzaldehyde, acetic acid, caproic acid, eugenol, furfural, over 150 other constituents, many of them traces.

Actions
Carminative, digestive, soothing.

Safety
Generally held to be non-toxic, non-irritant and non-sensitising.

Principal Uses

Physical:
- » Indigestion
- » Compulsive eating

Behavioural:
- » Moody animals, especially females
- » Bitterness of heart

Think "Vanilla" for:
Moody mares, especially if their moods are cyclical and they have a bitter attitude towards the world and/or there is a connection with the digestive system

VETIVER

(Vetiveria Zizanoides)

Element: Earth (Water)

History and Character:
A tall tropical grass with scented tufts and a spreading root system. Native to Southern India (where it is known as the Oil of Tranquillity), Indonesia and Sri Lanka, it is now mostly cultivated in Java, Haiti and Reunion. Traditionally, Indians have used vetiver as a vermin repellent for their animals and woven into aromatic matting for their houses. The Indians also anoint themselves with the oil in Hot Season to help keep them cool, and in Ayurveda it is used for joint problems and eczema. Energetically, vetiver is nurturing, the 'Earth mother' oil, calming and reassuring; it is grounding and helps to bring us back into the present, gathering scattered energies. I call it the 'Labrador' oil as I commonly use it for the over-enthusiastic 'love me, love me,' behaviour that is typical of Labrador retriever dogs. Conversely, it is also useful for underweight animals who are apologetic about their existence.

Synonyms
Andropogon Muricatus, Khus Khus, Vetivert.

Cultivation/sustainability
Cultivated. No issues

Extraction and Characteristics
Steam distillation of the roots and rootlets. The oil is viscous and dark amber.

Fragrance
Smoky, wet earth, with sweet overtones.

Principal Constituents

Alcohols: vetiverol

Ketones: β-vetivone, α-vetivone

Sesquiterpenes: α-murolene, vetivene, α-copaene, unresolved mixture C15 H22, unr

---

Vetiver for tranquility

Courtesy of Sherri Cappabianca, Animal PsychAromaticist, animal acupressure massage practitioner.

Samantha ("Sammie") is a hound mix, probably about a year and a half old when I saw her. In her young life she had been bounced around through several homes and rescue organizations, and had her name changed a couple of times before winding up at what looks to be her forever home. As a result, she had terrible separation anxiety. Whenever her people left home or even left the room and closed the door behind, she would start to bark and howl, escalating to the point where it was so loud the neighbours believed she was being physically harmed. This would continue until they returned home. Her people tried everything they could think of and finally called me in to help. I selected three oils for her, cedarwood, vetiver and violet leaf. When I visited their home and showed them how to offer the oils, Sammie took a particular liking to the vetiver, which was diluted 2 drops in 5 ml of St.John's wort carrier oil. She wouldn't leave the bottle alone! Vetiver is a grounding oil, nurturing, calming and reassuring. It helps animals who are emotionally insecure or those who seek constant reassurance. After licking the bottle and the oil on my hand, she lay down next to the bottle and continue to inhale, relaxing deeply. Almost immediately after this her people began to notice a change in her. She seemed calmer and they were able to leave the room without Sammie panicking. Soon thereafter, they were able to leave the home with no barking. Today, Sammie still has some separation anxiety issues, but they are minor.

Actions

Anti-anaemic, antiseptic, circulatory tonic, emmenagogic, glandular tonic (pancreatic secretion), immunostimulant.

Safety

Generally held to be non-toxic, non-irritant and non-sensitising.

Principal Uses

Physical:
- » Physically run down
- » Underweight for no good reason
- » Anaemia

Behavioural:
- » Ungrounded animals who don't know where they begin and end

- » Emotional insecurity
- » Perfectionists
- » Restlessness
- » Pushy animals who try to walk all over you

Think "Vetiver" for:

Animals who walk all over you in enthusiasm or fear, or don't know where their feet are and tend to knock things over or step on you and seek constant reassurance.

VIOLET LEAF

(Viola Odorata)

Element: Fire (Water)

History and Character

A low growing, spreading perennial with dark green heart-shaped leaves, violet flowers and a tuberous root. Violet leaf is native to Europe and can be found growing in shady protected areas. It was cultivated as far back as 400BC by the Greeks and has a long history of use as a medicine, mostly for congestive heart conditions and capillary fragility of the skin. British herbalists use both flower and leaf for eczema and skin eruptions, particularly when associated with rheumatic symptoms. Energetically, violet leaf is grounding and settling, giving the strength of heart to move on from situations where energy is caught in a pattern of mistrust.

Synonyms

Heartsease, Sweet Violet, English Violet

Cultivation/sustainability

Cultivated. No known issues

Extraction and Characteristics

Solvent extraction from the fresh leaves. The resulting absolute is a thick viscous green product with a tendency to crystallise. There is also an absolute produced from the flowers.

Fragrance

A green herby, odour reminiscent of fresh cucumbers and a slightly floral undertone.

Principal Constituents
Alcohols: dodecanol, hexanol, octen-4-ol, heptadienol, nonadienol, benzyl alcohol
Aldehydes: nonadienal, pentadecenal

Actions
Analgesic (mild), anti-inflammatory, antirheumatic, antiseptic, decongestant (liver), diuretic, expectorant, laxative, soporific, stimulant (circulatory).

Safety
Generally held to be non-toxic, non-irritant and non-sensitising.

Principal Uses
Physical:
- » Old animals with aches and pains and a loss of self confidence
- » Chronic pain
- » Arthritis

Behavioural:
- » Loss of trust in themselves or others
- » New home
- » Bargy, flighty animals that spook easily

Think 'Violet leaf' for:
Insecure animals who try to hide their insecurity through 'loud' behaviour or when a change in environment or a traumatic incident has caused a change in behaviour.
Old animals in chronic pain, suffering silently.

YARROW

(Achillea Millefolium)

Element: Wood (Water)

History and Character
Yarrow is a perennial herb growing up to 1 metre/3 ft high. It has a basal rosette of fern-like leaves and a tall stem bearing a tight-knit cluster of white to pale pink flowers that look like a shield, protection being one of its signatures. Native to Eurasia and found in hedgerows throughout Britain it has naturalised in most temperate zones but the chamazulene content is highest in the oil distilled in Eastern Europe. It has been used since ancient times and was reputed to have been used by Achilles (hence the name) for wounds caused by iron weapons. The stalks are traditionally used for reading the I-Ching. Yarrow helps release energy held around physical and emotional scars and past trauma, especially when the trauma manifests as angry fear. Yarrow is one of the essential oils I use most commonly for animals, especially troubled animals with an unknown history, or if I suspect past trauma of any kind because of behaviours or scars.

Synonyms
Soldier's wort, Milfoil, Nosebleed, Old Man's Pepper, and many other local variations.

Cultivation/sustainability
Cultivated mostly. No issues

Extraction and Characteristics
Steam distillation of the dried herb. The oil varies from pale green to a deep blue depending on chamazulene content, the bluer the oil the more anti-inflammatory it is.

Fragrance
Sweet, herbaceous, spicy, with a soft woody dryout.

Principal Constituents
Terpenes: β-farnesene, α-farnesene, α-humulene, ρ-cymene, camphene, α-pinene, caryophyllene, chamazulene
Alcohols: borneol
Aldehydes: neral
Ketones: camphor, thujone, artemisia ketone
Esters: bornyl acetate
Oxides:1,8 cineole, bisabolol oxide. bisabolone oxide

Actions
Anti-allergenic, anti-inflammatory, antiseptic, antispasmodic, carminative, expectorant, febrifuge, haemostatic, hypotensive.

Safety
Generally held to be non-toxic, non-irritant and non-sensitising. One of the few oils you can use undiluted. Avoid in pregnancy and young children. Occasionally yarrow can trigger 'acting out' of a past trauma the first time it is given.

Principal Uses
Physical:
  » Wounds
  » Inflammations
  » Sprains and strains
  » Urinary infections
  » Ear infections
  » Allergies
  » Skin problems of all kinds
  » Arthritis
  » Scars
Behavioural:
  » Emotional release around scars
  » Fearful anger
  » Past abuse

Think 'Yarrow' for:
Any animal whose past history is unknown to you, especially if it is exhibiting behavioural problems, or if there is a history of physical or emotional trauma.

YLANG-YLANG

(Cananga Odorata)

Element: Fire

History and Character

Ylang Ylang is a tall tropical tree with large shiny leaves and fragrant tender flowers that can be pink or yellow. The yellow flowers are considered best for essential oil. Ylang ylang is native to tropical Asia and the major oil producers are in Madagascar, Reunion and the Comoro Islands. In Indonesia the flowers are spread on the beds of newlyweds; it has also been used to encourage hair growth, to combat fever (including malaria) and fight infections. Energetically, it is a deeply calming oil, slowing heart rate and breathing and helping in situations where emotions overwhelm reason. It is similar to jasmine in its uses but better suited to young animals, especially when they are on the cusp of adulthood and finding their place in the pack/ herd hierarchy.

Synonyms

Unona Odorantissimum, Flower of Flowers.

Cultivation/sustainability

Mostly cultivated. No issues

Extraction and Characteristics

Steam distillation of the freshly picked flowers. The first hour of distillation produces what is known as ylang ylang extra, which is of a superior quality. Ylang ylang 1, 2 and complete are considered inferior. The oil is a pale yellowish liquid.

Fragrance

Intensely sweet floral, balsamic, spicy.

Principal Constituents

Alcohols: linalol
Terpenes: germacrene D, β-caryophellene, γ-cadinene, δ-cadinene
Ethers: ρ-cresyl methyl ether
Esters: benzyl benzoate, geranyl acetate, methyl salicylate, benzyl acetate, farnesyl acetate

Actions

Antidepressant, antiseptic, aphrodisiac, euphoric, hypotensive, sedative and tonic.

Safety

Generally held to be non-toxic, non-irritant and non-sensitising.

Henry the humble beagle

Henry was an 18-month old beagle who was bred to show. He was a nice looking young dog, very polite and well-behaved, however he kept losing marks in the show ring because when the judge looked him over he lowered his tail. Dogs lower their tails to show submission and Henry was just trying to be polite to this large person who was leaning over him in a way that seems aggressive to dogs. I explained this to the owner but I also agreed to try and find an oil to help Henry feel happier with the situation. Ylang ylang boosts self-confidence and 'joie de vivre' and Henry loved the oil. I diluted 1 drop in 5 ml of hemp seed base oil and he sniffed it keenly twice a day for three days before losing interest. His owner thought Henry was carrying himself with more confidence and was more responsive and playful. The week after that Henry went to a show. He was offered the oil before entering the ring, but wasn't very interested. When the judge went over him Henry's tail stayed high and proud, and he won the class.

Principal Uses

Physical:
  » Tachycardia
  » Hyperpnoea
  » Hair growth

Behavioural:
  » Sexual anxiety
  » Stereo-typical behaviours
  » Young animals who lack self confidence

Think 'Ylang-ylang' for:

Young animals who are nervous, restless, or lack confidence, especially if it is related to hierarchical problems, or there is any hair loss.

CARRIER OIL PROFILES (MA4)

Below are detailed descriptions of a selection of vegetable and macerated herbal oils commonly used for diluting essential oils for animals. There are many more vegetable oils available, however I have limited myself to those I use most often with animals. It is not essential to have a choice of carrier oils, you can easily manage with one good neutral carrier, such as sunflower. However using the precise carrier oil your animal needs in any given situation is beneficial. And sometimes animals just want a herbal oil.

*M denotes a macerated oil.

CALENDULA *M

Calendula Officinalis

Element: Earth (Fire)

History and Character
Calendula, also known as marigold, is a cheerful presence in gardens across the globe. It grows easily in any soil and is reputed to help keep vegetables free from pests, so is used as a companion plant in the vegetable patch. The double-orange flowers are the best ones to use for macerating and the oil takes on their beautiful golden colour. Calendula is a valuable healer, and as it is hard to find a good quality essential oil from this plant, the macerated oil is particularly useful. I use it often as a carrier oil and as a food supplement for stomach problems.

Synonym
Marigold oil (caution: oil of Tagetes glandulifera is also known as marigold, so check the Latin name when purchasing this oil).

Therapeutic uses
Internally it can be used for:

» Ulcers
» Indigestion
» Gall bladder complaints
» Hormonal problems

Externally it is one of the best skin healers we know, especially useful for:

» Slow healing wounds
» Bruises and capillary damage
» Lymphoedema
» Fungal infections
» Irritations

Emotional energy
Uplifting, cheerful, comforting.

Cautions
No known contraindications, do not confuse with oil from Tagetes patula.

CARROT OIL *M

Daucus Carota. L ssp Sativus

Element: Earth (Wood)

History and Character

Macerated carrot oil is made from the familiar orange root found in most kitchens. This carrier oil is a wonderful complement to carrot seed essential oil, especially in cases of poor skin or hoof condition. The oil is a rich orange colour, which is sometimes used as a food colouring and will stain white fur. It is rich in beta-carotene, vitamins A, B, C, D, E and F.

Therapeutic uses

» Tonic to the skin and hooves
» Helps heal damaged skin including scar tissue
» Soothing for itchy skin and eczema
» Helps repair old damaged skin
» Very nourishing, useful when animals are run down

Emotional energy

Strengthening, nourishing.

Cautions

Ingestion of excessive amounts of carrots or carrot juice can result in hypervitaminosis which causes yellowing of the skin and mucous membranes and progressive flakiness of the skin. You must also watch for 'imitation' carrot oil, which is made by adding carotene or other colorants to a base oil.

COMFREY OIL *M

Symphytum officinale

Element: Wood (Water)

History and Character

Comfrey's large hairy leaves and delicate purplish-pink flowers are a common sight throughout Europe, but especially in the British Isles. The macerated oil can be made from the roots or leaves of this sturdy plant, or both. Comfrey is a well-known healer's plant having been used extensively in herbal medicine. One of the common names of comfrey is Knitbone because of its ability to speed the healing of broken bones, bruises and wounds. It was also traditionally used for irritable coughs and chronic lung conditions.

Therapeutic uses

» Traumatic injury
» Broken bones
» Scar tissue and proud flesh

» Bruised emotions and long running emotional wounds that are simmering below the surface
» Strengthens the lungs

Emotional energy
Heals past hurt, helps to move on, strengthening.

Cautions
Do not use on puncture wounds or other very deep wounds as it is possible to speed the healing too much so the wound closes before it is clear of infection deeper down. Over-consumption of the root has caused cancer in mice.

GRAPESEED OIL

Vitis Vinifera

Element: Metal

History and Character
Grapeseed is probably the finest and lightest of oils, so useful as a neutral base oil. It is also colourless, almost odourless and hypoallergenic with no strongly active therapeutic properties of its own. This makes it an excellent carrier for essential oils when treating emotional/behavioural problems.

Therapeutic uses

» A neutral base oil for emotional problems. It is easily digestible and leaves the skin smooth without being greasy.

Emotional energy
Neutral, penetrative.

Caution
None known

HEMP SEED OIL

Cannabis Sativa

Element: Water

History and Character

Hemp seed oil is extracted from the seeds of the cannabis plant. The oil does not contain the psychoactive properties, but it is relaxing, warming and comforting. It has a strong nutty flavour, a high gamma linoleic acid (GLA) content and is nutritionally high in protein. The same plant is used for making a strong, pliable material or rope and Hemp seed oil is a great carrier oil for animals who are having a hard time 'holding it together', physically or emotionally.

Therapeutic uses

» It has been used successfully in the treatment of eczema
» Possible benefits for degenerative diseases
» Grounding and comforting
» Behavioural problems, especially anxiety related
» General weakness physically
» Arthritis

Emotional energy

Warming, gives security, grounding, relaxing.

Caution

None known.

HYPERICUM (ST JOHN'S WORT) *M

Hypericum Perforatum

Element: Fire (Wood)

History and Character

Hypericum oil is an amazing blood-red colour due to the presence of hypericin, an effective antiviral agent. It is made by soaking buds and flowers in (preferably) olive oil. In olden times this plant was thought to protect against evil spirits, something often said of plants that are now known to have a strong psychological effect; St John's wort is often used as a natural substitute for Prozac. Knights used it on sword wounds and it is now scientifically proven to be antibacterial and beneficial to wounds where there is nerve damage.

Therapeutic uses

- » Depression
- » Inflamed nerve conditions, such as sciatica
- » Burns
- » Skin inflammations
- » Wounds
- » Bruises
- » Arthritis
- » Extreme nervousness
- » Unpredictable moods

Emotional energy
Balancing, soothing, cooling.

Caution
Ingestion of high doses of hypericum can cause photo-sensitisation in light-skinned animals.

JOJOBA OIL (WAX)

Simmondsia Sinensis

Element: Water (Metal)

History and Character
The jojoba plant is native to the deserts of southwest USA; it is a small leathery plant that takes 12 years to reach maturity and can be planted to prevent arid land becoming desert. The plant does not, strictly speaking, produce oil, but wax, which is highly stable, remaining unchanged for a period of years. It has very little odour and is nourishing to the skin. I use it most often as a neutral carrier oil for emotional problems.

Therapeutic uses

- » Almost all skin problems
- » Hair conditioner
- » Anti-inflammatory
- » Arthritis and rheumatism
- » Possible appetite suppressant

Emotional energy
Neutral, smooth.

Cautions
Jojoba oil fed to rats caused changes to histological and enzymatic activity. Do not use as a food supplement. Contact dermatitis has been reported.

NEEM SEED OIL

Azadirachta indica

Element: Metal

History and Character

The neem tree is known in India as 'the village pharmacy'. For more than 4,500 years traditional healers have used the neem bark, seeds, leaves, fruit, gum and oils for dozens of internal and external medical treatments. The most common historical uses of neem were for treatment of skin diseases, inflammation, fevers and as an antiparasitic. In India it is claimed to be contraceptive. Neem oil is effective against at least 200 insects. It is apparently so distasteful that most insects won't eat a plant treated with it, but if they do, it disrupts their hormones, fatally preventing the bugs from shedding their outgrown skins.

Therapeutic uses

- » Rheumatism and arthritis
- » Eczema
- » Ringworm
- » Scabies
- » Fly and flea sprays

Emotional energy

Cooling, clarifying, sharp.

Caution

Although the hormonal effect shown on insects has not been seen to affect mammals, do not use in pregnancy.

OLIVE OIL

Olea Europaea

Element: Fire (Wood)

History and Character

The olive tree has been part of Western culture as a food and beauty aid for many centuries, the first record of its cultivation being 5,000 years ago. Native to the Mediterranean region, the tree is a symbol of prosperity and peace. The tree is slow growing, to a height of about 8 metres/26 ft maximum, producing fruit after 15 years and living for centuries. The oil is extracted from the flesh of the fruit, the first pressing is called virgin, and the first portion of this pressing is called extra virgin and is the best quality oil. Olive oil is calming, demulcent and emollient and contains a component (oleocanthal) which works like the anti-inflammatory ibuprofen.

Therapeutic uses

- » Stimulates bile secretion
- » Mildly anti-inflammatory
- » Skin soothing
- » Lowers blood pressure
- » Laxative
- » Highly nutritive

Emotional energy:
Nourishing and strengthening, peaceful.

Caution
May cause sensitisation when applied topically. Do not use 'commercial' olive oil.

PASSIONFLOWER *M

Passiflora Incarnata

Element: Fire

History and Character
Passiflora is a fast growing perennial vine native to the southern hemisphere. The plant is named for the passion of Christ due to the shape of its stigma and stamens, which are said to represent the 'Instruments of Torture' used in the Crucifixion of Christ. There is an expressed oil made from the seeds, which is used in the food and cosmetic industry. The best oil for use with animals is that produced by macerating flowers in organic sunflower oil. The oil is soothing and sedative and particularly useful for stress-related behavioural problems in dogs.

Therapeutic uses

- » Sedative
- » Antispasmodic
- » Nervous excitability
- » Heart irregularities

Emotional energy
Relaxing, supportive.

Caution
None known.

SESAME OIL

Sesamum Indicum

Element: Earth

History and Character

Sesame oil is a stable antioxidant oil. It is almost odourless and high in vitamins A, B and E, calcium, magnesium and phosphorous. It has natural sun-protective qualities and is a free-radical scavenger. I use it for nervous animals or those who seem underweight or insecure in themselves.

Therapeutic uses

- » Improves blood platelet count, so is good for anaemia when taken internally
- » Spleen disorders
- » Soothing to the digestive tract
- » A mild laxative
- » Dry skin and broken veins

Emotional energy

Warming, strengthening, energising.

Caution

Possible hypersensitisation.

SUNFLOWER OIL

Helianthus Anuus L

Element: Metal (All)

History and Character

Sunflower oil is another of the 'neutral' oils, as it is essentially odourless. Because there is so much commercial production of sunflower oil it is really important to buy organic cold-pressed oil. If I were only allowed to have one carrier oil, this would be it.

Therapeutic uses

- » A neutral carrier oil for emotional problems
- » Skin ulcers
- » Bruises
- » Rhinitis and sinusitis

Emotional energy

Neutral, supportive.
Caution: none known

HYDROSOL PROFILES (MA5)

Following are profiles of a selection of hydrosols. In this section I highlight any differences between the hydrosol and essential oil and how I use them. You can always replace any essential oil with its hydrosol, so for more detailed information about what each hydrosol can do, refer to the essential oil profiles (MA3).

ANGELICA ROOT

(Angelica Archangelica)

Characteristics
Angelica root hydrosol has a sweet, rooty fragrance with a hint of river bottom or wet earth. It is sweeter and easier to accept than the essential oil and I find it delicious.

Therapeutic uses
I have found this water to be very protective and grounding with a light-hearted quality to it. Physically it is a great digestive and a useful liver tonic and mildly sedative. I use it much more on a physical level than I do the oil.

Stability
Medium to high.

Caution
Treat as phototoxic.

CARROT SEED

(Daucus Carota)

Characteristics
The fragrance of this hydrosol is very similar to the essential oil but much milder, like a good carrot soup, sweet, warm, earthy and nourishing.

Therapeutic uses
Carrot seed is diuretic and cleanses and supports both the liver and gall bladder making it very useful for detoxification e.g. in food related skin allergies in dogs. It is also indicated for colitis as it soothes smooth muscle, and is said to encourage beneficial flora. Because of its cell reparative properties it is useful for any damaged skin and unlike the oil, which can be irritant, it is very soothing to the skin.

Stability
High.

Cautions
None known.

CHAMOMILE, ROMAN

(Chamamaelum Nobile)

Characteristics
Chamomile hydrosol smells very similar to high quality oil but with softer overtones. I find it one of the more robust of the waters with a more grounding effect than the oil. It tastes like a rich chamomile tea.

Therapeutic uses
Chamomile hydrosol is excellent for soothing upset tummies and tempers and even better for those of a delicate nature. It is great for bathing gunky eyes and any irritated skin conditions, although do not use it long term on very dry skin.

Stability
High.

Cautions
Can be drying to the skin if used long term.

CORNFLOWER

(Centaurea Cyanus)

Characteristics
There is no essential oil of cornflower so this hydrosol is particularly useful. The fragrance is fresh and intriguing, quite sharp, with a slightly lemony/green edge.

Therapeutic uses
Cornflower is one of the best choices for irritated eyes and can be used as an eyewash. It's anti-haematoma, so a good choice for bumps and bruises, and it can be used to wash out wounds without irritating sensitive tissue. Cornflower hydrosol hydrates tissue, and can be used as a hair conditioner. Also use to reduce fever and as a general tonic especially for the liver.

Stability
Low to moderate.

Cautions
Do not use in pregnancy.

DILL

(Anethum Graveolens)

Characteristics
Dill hydrosol smells like the fresh herb with a slightly musty undertone and a sweet top note; it tastes green and fresh especially when diluted.

Therapeutic uses
Dill is really soothing to the digestive tract (its name comes from the Norse 'Dylla', to soothe) and is great for spasmodic pain, especially of the digestive tract. Dill is useful for colic, irritable bowel syndrome, and dogs with smelly breath. It could also be used for poor lactation. I use it where I would use fennel essential oil.

Stability
High.

Cautions
None known.

EUCALYPTUS

(Eucalyptus Globulus)

Characteristics
The smell of eucalyptus hydrosol is sweet and much lighter and less penetrating than the essential oil, but to my nose has a slightly sickly undertone. The taste is sharp and tingly with a distinctly green flavour. It is drying, both topically and energetically.

Therapeutic uses
I use it in fly sprays although not on sensitive or damaged skin as it is rather drying and can sting. It is a strong immune stimulant and useful for bringing down fevers. Spray liberally around stables or kennels to inhibit the spread of infection and boost immune systems.

Stability
Medium to high.

Cautions
Do not apply to sensitive skin.

FRANKINCENSE

(Boswellia Carterii)

Characteristics

The scent of frankincense hydrosol is slightly sweeter than the oil, but softer and thicker, closer to the smell of incense, albeit with a slightly bitter edge. The taste is quite bitter when undiluted but much more palatable when diluted.

Therapeutic uses

As with the oil, frankincense is a great hydrosol for fearful fretting and asthmatic conditions and I find it more comforting than the oil. It can be used as a rinse for mouth and gum infections. It can also be used in gels for irritated skin as it hydrates dry skin.

Stability

Medium to high.

Cautions

None known.

GERANIUM

(Pelargonium Graveolens)

Characteristics

The fragrance of geranium hydrosol is sweetly floral, rich green and slightly lemon with only a touch of the musty undertones of the oil.

Therapeutic uses

Geranium hydrosol is the best general balancer whenever the body/mind has gone to one extreme or another. Anti-inflammatory and cooling to the skin I use it often in older females who itch chronically. It can be used on wounds to stop bleeding, or on scabs to relieve itching and help the skin heal well.

Stability

Low.

Cautions

None known.

GINGER ROOT

(Zingiber Officinalis)

Characteristics
Ginger hydrosol has a wonderful earthy aroma, warm and sharp. The taste is almost too earthy undiluted and a little hot, but diluted well it is pleasant and warming.

Therapeutic uses
Ginger boosts self-confidence and gives a feeling of 'can do'. It is also a good digestive stimulant and very warming for the whole body, good for colds and chills. These circulatory stimulating and warming properties make ginger hydrosol a very comforting rub or spray for older arthritic animals.

Stability
Medium to high.

Cautions
Unknown.

JUNIPER BERRY

(Juniperis Communis)

Characteristics
Juniper berry hydrosol has a musty, woody fragrance yet with a delicate sweetness. It is very astringent and uncomfortably drying when undiluted.

Therapeutic uses
This hydrosol is a powerful diuretic, supportive of kidney function and a good circulatory stimulant, use it topically to ease tired muscles after a workout. I use it mostly as a psychic protector and cleanser, useful for those who get overwhelmed in crowds, in which case I put it in a spray bottle and spray through the aura of the animal.

Stability
Low.

Cautions
Do not use in pregnancy and kidney disease.

IMMORTELLE

(Helicrysum Angustifolium or Stoechas)

Characteristics

Sharp and sweet, with an undertone of curry, the fragrance of this tough little plant fills the air on warm days. The plant is a small shrub with feathery pale green leaves and bright yellow flowers, that retain their fragrance even when dried. Hence the name 'immortelle' or 'everlast'. It grows in dry, rocky terrain on south facing slopes, brightening up what would otherwise be barren slopes.

Therapeutic Uses:

This hydrosol is a first aid in a bottle. Use it to wash wounds or soak cotton to use as a poultice on bruises and sprains. It also soothes itchy skin, especially allergic reactions. It is good for grumpy "liverish" behaviour as it smoothes Liver qi.
Bright and cheerful against all odds, uplifting, energising.

Stability:

High.

Cautions:

None known

LAVENDER

(Lavandula Angustifolia)

Characteristics

Lavender hydrosol smells exactly as we expect the plant to smell (which isn't always the case with hydrosols), sweet and woody, with a robust middle note of honey; rounder but less complex than a good lavender oil.

Therapeutic uses

I mainly use lavender hydrosol for its soothing properties on irritated skin and sunburn and to help in the recovery of damaged skin. It is also a good space-spray for places where there is a lot of anxiety and nervousness, such as kennels, vet clinics and shows; it is comforting yet not too intrusive.

Stability

High.

Cautions

None known.

LEMON BALM

(Melissa Officinalis)

Characteristics
Lemon balm (or melissa) hydrosol has a light, sweet, citrus-green fragrance, very refreshing and uplifting with a sharp edge. Diluted in water it is fresh and uplifting.

Therapeutic uses
The hydrosol of lemon balm is not as strong an immune stimulant as the essential oil, but still useful. I use it for calming nerves as it is very relaxing without being sedative. In humans, it has been used successfully for ADHD, reducing hyperactivity and increasing focus. Lemon balm is a good digestive aid. Use in moderation.

Stability
Moderate.

Cautions
Hypotension.

LENTISK/MASTIC

(Pistacia lentiscus)

Characteristics:
Also known as wild pistachio, this shrub grows on rocky hillsides throughout the mediterranean basin. It is a bright, cheerful bush with small rubbery leaves. Its name derives from the Greek word "To chew" because it was the original chewing gum and has a strong affinity with dental health.

TherapeuticUses:
I have included this slightly obscure aromatic because it is so useful in dental health. It has a powerful antibacterial action but is very well tolerated by all animals as a mouthwash. I add it to a bowl of water for cats to self-clean. It is also anti-inflammatory and soothing to the digestive system. Emotionally invigorating, it gives you strength and clears out stagnant energies, but is at the same time grounding.

Stability:
Medium.

Cautions:
None known

NEROLI (ORANGE BLOSSOM)

(Citrus Aurantium var. Amara)

Characteristics

Orange blossom hydrosol has an intensely floral fragrance with more of a detectable bitter edge than the oil; it is highly complex and much more easily assimilated when diluted.

Therapeutic uses

I use this hydrosol for calming hysterical fear, or any other situation where emotion has overcome the 'civilised mind'. Like the essential oil, the hydrosol steadies the heart physically and emotionally, so is great for shock or steadying the nerves before something stressful like travelling. Use for colic with gas or bloating. I have also used it internally as a support for itchy skin caused by food intolerance.

Stability

High.

Cautions

Hypotension, potentially drying to the skin.

PEPPERMINT

(Mentha Piperita)

Characteristics

This hydrosol is full of life with a wonderful fresh green, zingy fragrance which is softer and wider than most peppermint essential oils.

Therapeutic uses

Peppermint hydrosol is great for colitis, colic, IBS, flatulence and for cleansing the digestive tract. It clears the liver and Liver Heat, calming irritable moods and red skin. Use peppermint hydrosol for cooling off on a physical level, especially in case of heat stroke.

Stability

Low.

Cautions

Avoid alcohol or other intoxicants. Do not use with very young.

ROSE

(Rosa Damascena)

Characteristics
A rose is a rose is a rose and the hydrosol smells much like the essential oil, although slightly sweeter.

Therapeutic uses
Use rose hydrosol for balancing hormones in animals of all ages. It is a nourishing water for those who feel hard done by or whose hearts have closed due to poor treatment and the subsequent loss of trust. It is also astringent and cooling for the skin. Rose can also be used as an eye wash to soothe redness and irritation and is an emotionally nourishing pick-me-up for post-natal recovery.

Stability
High.

Cautions
Pregnancy, except after labour has started.

ROSEMARY

(Rosmarinus officinalis)

Characteristics
Rosemary hydrosol smells green and woody and almost floral; the taste is herbaceous and sharp undiluted, but quite sweet when diluted.

Therapeutic uses
Use rosemary hydrosol as a coat conditioning rinse after shampooing, it gives a shine and encourages healthy hair growth. Rosemary is a mental stimulant, so is good for those who can't focus, or seem vague or confused. It is also a hepatic stimulant and is good for those who have a tendency to gain weight or have slow digestion. It can be used after strenuous exercise to help rid the body of uric and lactic acid, likewise for arthritis. Also consider using it for respiratory distress, especially if allergy related. I have used it in a homeopathic solution to reduce seizures and fits.

Stability
Moderate to high.

Cautions
Do not use in case of high blood pressure or early pregnancy.

TEA TREE

(Melaleuca Alternifolia)

Characteristics

Tea tree hydrosol smells much like the essential oil but not as sharp and with subtle woody undertones. It tastes dry and medicinal and is not pleasant undiluted, but diluted it is quite invigorating and an excellent mouth wash.

Therapeutic uses

I mainly use this hydrosol as an antiseptic wound wash. It can also be added to fly or flea sprays, although it can be slightly drying to the coat. It is a good immune stimulant, and antiseptic internally and externally. Use undiluted as a foot soak for infected toenails. The hydrosol is better than the essential oil on an energetic level for protection of personal space and other Metal issues.

Stability

Medium to high.

Cautions

None known

THYME

(Thymus Vulgaris)

Characteristics

Thyme hydrosol has a warm, dry, herbaceous fragrance much like the plant at the height of summer. There is a difference in its characteristics according to chemotype, as with the oil.

Therapeutic uses:

Thyme is antibacterial, antiseptic and antifungal, a good wound wash, especially if the wound is oozing, but not if the area is very hot. Use thyme for dermal infections, especially if there is excessive moisture, and for bad breath arising from digestive problems.

Stability

High.

Cautions

Thyme can be a stimulant, don't use in the evening.

WITCH HAZEL

(Hamamelis Virginiana)

Characteristics
This is another hydrosol that has no equivalent essential oil, and is very useful in the first aid kit. A much more woody fragrance than the witch hazel we are used to from the chemist, which is not a hydrosol but a tincture in alcohol. I love this fragrance, it is delicate and enlivening.

Therapeutic uses
Nothing compares to witch hazel when it comes to healing broken capillaries and bruises. It is soothing for all types of skin complaints particularly eczema. It is also antiseptic and cicatrisant, so a useful wound wash; and calms agitation.

Stability
Unstable, short shelf life.

Cautions
Do not use commercially available witch hazel as it always contains alcohol. Not for internal use.

YARROW

(Achillea Millefolium)

Characteristics
The fragrance of yarrow hydrosol is much more woody than the oil but with similar hay-like overtones and an edge of bitterness.

Therapeutic uses
Yarrow hydrosol is a soothing wash for irritated skin and allergic reactions, also for wounds as it helps to stem bleeding. It is also good for digestive problems especially constipation. It is antispasmodic for both digestive and reproductive systems, good for mares who get tight back muscles when in season, or for bitches who feel depressed and moody. It can also be used as an anti-inflammatory compress, especially for excess fluid.

Stability
High.

Cautions
Do not use in pregnancy.

ESSENTIAL OILS FOR SPECIFIC MERIDIANS (MA6)

This chart lists essential oils that are particularly suited to specific meridian systems, for those of you who practice Chinese medicine.

	CONCEPTION VESSEL	GOVERNING VESSEL	STOMACH	SPLEEN-PANCREAS	HEART	SMALL INTESTINE	BLADDER	KIDNEY	HEART PROTECTOR	TRIPLE WARMER	GALL BLADDER	LIVER	LUNG	LARGE INTESTINE
Angelica Root	X		X	X				X	X	X		X		
Basil (sweet)	X		X		X								X	
Benzoin Resinoid	X	X	X	X									X	
Bergamot	X				X			X				X		
Cajeput	X								X				X	
Carrot Seed			X		X						X	X		X
Cedarwood Atlas	X	X					X	X	X				X	
Chamomile German			X	X							X	X	X	X
Chamomile Roman	X		X							X	X	X		
Chastetree	X	X			X	X		X		X				
Cistus	X				X	X		X					X	X
Clary Sage	X	X						X					X	
Cypress	X			X				X					X	X
Elemi	X										X		X	
Eucalyptus				X									X	X
Fennel, Sweet	X		X	X				X						
Flouve/hay	X			X									X	X
Frankincense	X		X								X		X	X
Garlic			X		X								X	X
Geranium	X			X	X			X	X	X	X			
Ginger		X	X	X	X		X	X	X				X	
Grapefruit			X	X							X	X		
Helichrysum	X	X			X							X	X	X
Hemp	X	X	X								X	X	X	X

	CONCEPTION VESSEL	GOVERNING VESSEL	STOMACH	SPLEEN-PANCREAS	HEART	SMALL INTESTINE	BLADDER	KIDNEY	HEART PROTECTOR	TRIPLE WARMER	GALL BLADDER	LIVER	LUNG	LARGE INTESTINE
Lavender	X		X	X	X	X				X	X	X		
Lavender green			X	X	X								X	
Lemon	X		X	X	X	X		X		X			X	
Lemongrass	X			X		X			X		X		X	
Lentisk		X	X									X	X	X
Manuka		X		X									X	X
Marjoram, Sweet		X	X	X					X					X
Melissa	X		X	X	X				X	X				
Myrrh	X		X			X							X	X
Neroli	X		X		X					X		X		
Nutmeg	X		X	X	X					X	X			
Orange, Sweet	X		X		X					X	X	X		
Patchouli	X	X	X	X				X	X					
Peppermint	X		X								X	X	X	X
Plai		X							X				X	X
Rhododendron	X				X				X	X			X	X
Ravensara	X	X											X	
Rosalina				X									X	
Rose	X				X				X	X		X		
Rosemary	X		X	X	X					X			X	
Seaweed							X	X	X	X	X	X		X
Spearmint			X	X									X	X
Tansy	X											X	X	X
Tea Tree													X	
Thyme	X		X	X				X		X			X	
Valerian Root	X		X	X	X			X		X				
Vanilla	X		X	X					X					
Vetiver	X		X	X				X	X	X				
Violet Leaf	X		X		X				X	X	X			
Yarrow	X	X					X	X	X			X	X	
Ylang-ylang	X				X	X			X					

INDEX OF THERAPEUTIC ACTIONS (MA7)

Therapeutic Action (MA7)	Juniper Berry	Jasmine	Hyssop	Hemp	Helichrysum	Grapefruit	Ginger	Geranium	Garlic	Frankincense	Flouve	Fennel, Sweet	Eucalyptus	Elemi	Cypress	Clary Sage	Cistus	Chastetree	Chamomile, Roman	Chamomile, German	Cedarwood	Carrot Seed	Cajeput	Bergamot	Benzoin	Basil (French)	Angelica Root
Analgesic	×	×			×		×	×		×	×		×						×		×	×					×
anthelmintic/vermifuge					×																			×	×		
Anti-Allergic/histamine					×																×						
Anti-Anaemic																											
Anti-Arthritic																											
Anti-Bacterial					×		×	×					×	×		×		×						×		×	×
Anti-Catarrhal					×		×			×			×					×			×						
Anti-Coagulant					×																						
Anti-Convulsant																											
Anti-Depressant/euphoric				×									×						×					×		×	
Anti-Diabetic	×				×			×																			
Anti-Emetic					×																						
Anti-Fungal					×			×					×			×				×				×			×
Anti-Infectious							×			×			×			×		×	×	×							×
Anti-Inflammatory					×			×					×			×			×	×	×				×		×
Anti-Lactogenic																											
Anti-Oxidant													×					×				×					
Anti-Parasitic																×		×			×						
Anti-Rheumatic						×												×		×							
Anti-Sclerotic																											
Anti-Septic	×				×	×		×						×			×	×			×	×		×			×
Anti-Spasmodic				×	×	×		×					×	×			×	×			×	×					×
Anti-Sudorific																	×	×									
Anti-Toxic																											×
Anti-Tussive																											
Anti-Viral					×		×							×							×			×		×	
Astringent							×		×		×															×	
Calmative/sedative				×									×				×	×		×	×						
Carminative				×			×	×					×					×			×	×		×		×	×
Cardio-Tonic					×																						
Cephalic																											×
Cholagogic/choleretic					×								×														
Cicatrizant/vulnerary				×	×	×	×	×			×			×			×		×	×				×	×		
Circulatory Stimulant					×								×														
Decongestant					×			×									×										
Detoxicant	×																×				×						
Digestive/stomachic	×				×		×	×		×			×			×		×	×	×							×
Diuretic	×				×				×				×			×		×		×				×			×
Emmenagogue																		×		×							
Expectorant					×				×				×			×		×			×	×		×	×		×
Febrifuge																					×	×		×			×
Haemostatic/styptic											×						×							×			
Hepatic/liver tonic																											
Hormone-Like													×			×	×		×								
Hypertensive				×																							
Hypotensive																											
Immune Tonic					×				×				×	×						×							
Insect Repellent											×				×							×					
Kidney tonic																											
Lactogen/galactagogue													×														×
Laxative													×														
Litholytic	×		×										×														
Lymphatic Stimulant	×								×															×			
Neurotonic																		×	×	×						×	×
Phlebotonic					×			×					×			×											
Regenerative																		×	×			×					
Respiratory Tonic													×								×						
Rubefacient														×							×						
Sexual Tonic				×					×																		
Stimulant					×								×							×	×						
Stomachic									×								×							×			
Sudorific																											
Tonic (general)					×		×	×	×				×							×		×	×	×			×
Uterine Tonic			×																								×
Vasodilator												×										×					

MA7-2	Ylang Ylang	Yarrow	Violet Leaf	Vetiver	Vanilla	Valerian Root	Thyme	Tea Tree	Tansy	Spearmint	Seaweed	Rosemary	Rose	Rosalina	Ravensara	Rhododendron	Peppermint	Plai	Patchouli	Orange (Sweet)	Nutmeg	Neroli	Myrrh	Melissa	Marjoram (sweet)	Manuka	Lentisk	Lemongrass	Lemon	Lavender, green	Lavender
Analgesic			×						×			×				×	×	×			×				×			×		×	×
anthelmintic/vermifuge							×											×													×
Anti-Allergic/histamine							×		×			×	×													×					×
Anti-Anaemic				×																									×		×
Anti-Arthritic												×																		×	×
Anti-Bacterial							×	×	×			×	×	×	×	×	×				×			×	×	×	×	×	×	×	×
Anti-Catarrhal												×						×													×
Anti-Coagulant												×										×						×			×
Anti-Convulsant																									×						×
Anti-Depressant/euphoric													×				×			×	×			×					×		
Anti-Diabetic	×																				×	×									
Anti-Emetic																				×		×									
Anti-Fungal								×	×			×					×			×				×	×	×	×	×	×	×	×
Anti-Infectious			×									×		×	×	×	×			×				×					×	×	×
Anti-Inflammatory		×	×						×			×	×	×	×	×	×	×		×				×	×			×	×	×	×
Anti-Lactogenic																	×														
Anti-Oxidant									×			×							×										×		
Anti-Parasitic							×																								
Anti-Rheumatic												×										×						×			
Anti-Sclerotic												×								×								×			
Anti-Septic		×	×						×								×				×	×	×	×		×	×	×	×	×	×
Anti-Spasmodic		×				×	×		×	×		×							×	×		×	×	×	×	×	×		×	×	×
Anti-Sudorific																×	×			×											
Anti-Toxic	×											×								×											
Anti-Tussive												×																	×		
Anti-Viral							×	×				×	×		×		×	×	×				×	×				×			
Astringent									×			×			×				×				×	×		×	×	×			
Calmative/sedative		×			×								×				×		×		×	×	×					×	×	×	×
Carminative				×	×	×	×		×			×							×		×	×	×	×				×			×
Cardio-Tonic	×											×										×	×								×
Cephalic																															
Cholagogic/choleretic												×									×										
Cicatrizant/vulnerary												×	×									×			×						×
Circulatory Stimulant			×	×																											×
Decongestant			×									×				×	×													×	
Detoxicant									×	×			×	×	×	×															
Digestive/stomachic				×	×							×	×							×	×		×	×	×	×			×		
Diuretic		×		×		×	×		×	×	×	×								×	×				×			×		×	
Emmenagogue			×									×										×									×
Expectorant		×	×				×	×	×	×				×	×		×		×			×	×	×			×		×	×	
Febrifuge							×	×	×						×					×	×										
Haemostatic/styptic		×											×																		
Hepatic/liver tonic		×								×	×		×							×			×								
Hormone-Like																	×			×						×					
Hypertensive							×					×					×														
Hypotensive		×					×					×	×						×							×					×
Immune Tonic				×							×						×			×		×	×						×		
Insect Repellent	×																	×					×			×		×	×		×
Kidney tonic		×					×					×	×																		
Lactogen/galactagogue																															
Laxative			×																	×											
Litholytic												×																×			
Lymphatic Stimulant																															
Neurotonic									×	×		×	×		×		×		×		×			×	×			×			
Phlebotonic										×									×		×							×			
Regenerative	×																														
Respiratory Tonic							×																			×					×
Rubefacient							×												×												
Sexual Tonic												×	×							×			×								
Stimulant							×				×	×	×							×											
Stomachic						×						×								×	×		×	×	×				×		
Sudorific																															
Tonic (general)									×	×		×							×			×	×	×							×
Uterine Tonic												×						×				×									
Vasodilator																										×					

CHAPTER 5

HOW TO MAKE NATURAL LOTIONS & POTIONS

Aren't we missing something?

It might seem strange to those of you familiar with massage as the primary method of delivering essential oils, that it has taken me this long to get to the subject of topical application.

I do have my reasons. Apart from the obvious logistical problems of covering a large fur-covered animal with oil, the truth is, most problems clear up if you reduce stress, provide a toxin-free diet and offer essential oils to lick or inhale.

In Western medicine it seems obvious that skin problems need topical application, but in Chinese medicine the skin is viewed as an early warning system. Systemic imbalances often make themselves known through the skin, only going deeper into the body if we do not pay attention. If we re-balance the whole system skin problems clear up. However there are times that a topical application can relieve pain or discomfort and speed up the healing process. Plus, making your own lotions and potions and natural bug repellents is fun!

Typical problems that call for topical application are:

- » Bacterial/fungal infection
- » Eczema
- » Sarcoids
- » Bruises/Strains
- » Arthritis
- » Flea/fly control

When using topicals you must still respect your animal's wishes. When you consider that most reported cases of adverse reaction to essential oils are due to topical use. Even animals who normally hate to have things rubbed into them will stand quietly, or move into your hand to make sure you get the right spot when allowed to choose their oils. When they no longer need the oils animals will fidget or move away as you try to apply the lotion.

Everyday items, such as fly spray, flea spray, or liniments, are also more effective when made for a specific animal, as each animal has a unique chemical make-up which affects the performance of all topical products. If you allow your animal to choose which oils it would like, the spray will work well and the animal will show no resistance to its application.

A word of caution! Use only hydrosols and base oils in topical applications for cats, NO ESSENTIAL OILS!

TOPICAL APPLICATIONS, STEP-BY-STEP

The protocol

Topical application should be used in conjunction with offering the oils to inhale because topical application alone is less effective. You need to assess the situation holistically and then make a short list of suitable oils, as per usual. Once you have made up the gel or clay as described below you will:

> » Offer essential oils separately in base oil as usual
>
> » Offer the gel to smell and apply it to the affected area
>
> » Watch the animal's reaction as you apply the gel and allow him/her to guide you in the application.

You will offer the oils and the gel before each application and once the animal loses interest in the oils, or expresses discomfort with the topical application discontinue use. You should then check to see if he needs other oils, or if he no longer needs the topical application.

GEL

I never use oil-based lotions or creams when working with animals. Apart from the fact that a dog covered in oily lotion is going to play havoc with your carpets, water-based gels and clays are easier to make at home.

Because essential oils do not like water but are attracted to lipids (fat), they move quickly out of the gel and into the animal's skin. This is especially relevant when working with dogs, as they will want to lick themselves clean sooner or later. If you use a water-based gel, by the time the dog cleans himself, the oil will have absorbed into his skin where you want it to be.

Interestingly, dogs do not usually lick the gel right off as one might expect, often leaving the gel/clay alone. If your dog does try to lick straight away, gently prevent him for five or 10 minutes. You can offer him the bottle of lotion to smell, or let him lick a little of the lotion from your hand while you are waiting.

I use gel when I want to soothe, encourage skin to heal and smooth, to moisten and soften skin or fur, for bruises, sprains, damaged tendons, and as a way to deliver essential oils rapidly into the skin for anti-inflammatory purposes. I also use gel as the base if I am going to dilute the mixture down to sprayable consistency, such as for fly and flea sprays, or add it to water as a wash to cover large areas.

Making a gel-based lotion, the quick method

To make a really basic gel, simply add essential oils to a shop-bought aloe vera gel or other water-based gel. This is quick, simple, and effective. You can also add a small amount of vegetable oil, if appropriate, to make a lightweight cream that dissolves easily into the skin and is not greasy on the fur. Good quality aloe vera gel can be bought in most health food shops or from aromatherapy suppliers, look for one that is free of additives, colouring and fragrance.

Making a gel based lotion, advanced method

You can also make your own gel from aloe juice or hydrosols as described in the next chapter, 'The Kitchen Pharmacy'. I like this method, because when we combine hydrosol, vegetable and essential oil we put the whole plant back together again, creating a unique synergy that a particular animal needs for healing.

Dilutions

The maximum suggested dilution for horses is 2%, for dogs 1%. For daily maintenance products, such as fly or flea spray, I add less essential oil. If I am dressing a wound I use more. I rely on the animal's preferences to guide how much of which oil I might add, as well as my knowledge of the essential oil's strength.

Divide the total drops of essential oils per gel between the selected oils, using more of the animal's favourite oil and less of oils that are harsh on the skin. For example, if you are using three oils for 100 ml of gel for a dog, your total is 20 drops and you might divide the oils 10-5-5, or 12-4-4 or 8-6-6.

Storage and safety

Gels and clays will keep for up to a year if refrigerated and kept free of bacterial contamination. All the utensils used for making gels and clays should be sterilised before use, as should the storage containers. Use latex gloves so you don't introduce bacteria with your fingers and to protect your hands from excessive doses of essential oil. And I highly recommend that you label and date every container as you fill it, so you don't end up with bottles full of unidentifiable potions of dubious vintage (bitter experience speaks!).

CLAYS

Did you ever wonder why your horse rolls in the muddiest spot in the field? Or your dog drinks from the muddiest puddle when they have lovely fresh water at home? They are just answering the calls of nature. Clay (mud) is a powerful healing agent and aids the body's healing processes. In the wild, animals use clay and mud for detoxification, as a cure for itchy skin, and to protect themselves from insect bites.

Essential oils can be added to clay and used where skin needs soothing or tightening; where there is oozing or weepy skin; to cool tendons and muscles; and to draw out abscesses. Clay creates a physical barrier against flies, midges and fungi, and in the case of fungi dries out the moisture they thrive on. Clay can also be used as a sunscreen. Or, add a little clay to water to create a source of natural minerals, plus help neutralise toxins and control worms.

Making lotions and potions

Essential oils: make a selection of oils for an animal to choose from, based on its life history, character and the current problem. As with any other treatment, choose oils to balance both the emotional and physical expression of the imbalance.

Vegetable oil: add up to 10% of the carrier oil the animal has chosen to the gel if appropriate.

Hydrosol: If you want to use a hydrosol gel as the base, offer the chosen hydrosol to the animal to make sure he agrees with your choice.

Blend the gel, using more drops of the essential oil the animal liked best and less of the ones he was moderately interested in.

Horses: Add a maximum of 2% essential oils (40 drops of essential oil=approx 2ml=2% of 100ml)

Dogs: add a maximum of 1% essential oils (20 drops =approx 1ml = 1% of 100ml)

Use higher dilutions (less oils) for sensitive, young, or old animals.

The colour of clay

There are several types of clay, generally classified and sold by colour; the colour reflecting the mineral content of the clay.

The clays I use most often are:

- » Green clay, strongly detoxifying and drawing, best for abscesses and for internal use
- » Kaolin clay, a light white clay, soothing for skin, skin stimulant, pH neutral
- » Bentonite clay, highly absorptive, skin protective and hydrating, helps soothe and strengthen the skin.

A couple of other useful clays that are harder to obtain are:

- » Yellow clay, exfoliating, stimulating and allows cellular oxygenation. It is known for its high power of oxygenation and relieving pain quickly
- » Red clay, stimulates circulation and strengthens the blood vessels, detoxifying.

Making mud pies

As with a gel, you can add essential oils, vegetable oil and hydrosol to clay and make it as thin or as thick as you need. If you want to draw infection from a wound or abscess make a thick paste; as a leg 'brace' for horses (to tone and stimulate tendons after work), add more liquid until the clay is the texture of double cream. Adding vegetable oil keeps the clay moist and pliable, which is good for sweet itch and mud-fever.

Safety

Clay can disrupt magnets so people with pacemakers should not use it. Clay should not be used in conjunction with any conventional medicines without professional advice.

SHAMPOOS

Personally, I suggest that you shampoo your animals as little as possible. A shiny, healthy, good smelling coat comes from within. If you feed your animal well and keep his stress levels low, your animal's coat will be the first to benefit. The main reason for scurfy, smelly or dull coats is poor diet and excess shampooing.

Shampoo strips the coat of natural oils and most coat conditioners are full of plastic or silicone, which give a superficial shine but ultimately damage the coat. However, if your dog has just rolled in fox faeces, or your horse had a mud bath before the show, you can add up to 25 drops of essential oil to 250 ml of unscented, SLS-free shampoo to make a purpose-built shampoo for horses or dogs. Most of the essential oil will rinse off with the water but a light fragrance will remain. Be aware that dogs have a lower skin pH than humans, so use shampoo made for dogs, oat-based is the gentlest. Or buy a natural bar soap.

FIRST AID

Essential oils should not be used instead of calling your vet, but can be used as an emergency medical kit for everyday mishaps. It is important to recognise when to call for veterinary assistance as it can make the difference between permanent lameness or worse. Generally speaking, if there is excessive bleeding or the possibility of a foreign object having entered the body, or there has been a strong impact that could have caused bone fractures or internal bleeding, or if your animal lost consciousness, call the vet. In all cases, "When in doubt, call the vet out". However, for situations you feel comfortable handling yourself, or while waiting for the vet to arrive, essential oils can help. Here are some suggestions for your first aid kit.

The 'essential' first aid kit

» Hydrosol of tea tree, helichrysum or thyme as a disinfectant wash.

» Essential oil of:

   » Yarrow – styptic, disinfectant, creates a protective barrier over the wound, anti-inflammatory, releases trauma.

   » Lavender – antiseptic, wound-healing, prevents scarring and proud flesh.

   » Helichrysum – antiseptic, anti-bruising, anti-inflammatory.

   » Neroli – for shock and colic.

   » Valerian- sedative.

   » Aloe vera gel – anti-inflammatory.

   » Calendula oil – anti-inflammatory, wound healing, anti-fungal, soothing.

   » Green clay – anti-toxicant, anti-inflammatory and cooling, draws out abscesses.

My cuts and wounds protocol

Wash with antiseptic hydrosol, or warm clean water with a teaspoon of sea salt. Liberal washing is advised.

Cover the wound with either yarrow, or make a yarrow hydrosol gel (see below) and add a few drops of tea tree or Rosalina.

Once the wound has started to heal cleanly, apply lavender undiluted or in a gel with cistus, this will speed repair, reduce scarring and prevent development of proud flesh.

THE KITCHEN PHARMACY

Natural solutions for common problems

Following are a few recipes for specific problems. I give you a selection of different oils with similar actions for each 'slot' in the recipe so your animal has choices. The most effective blends all have a harmonious fragrance, with no single essential oil standing out too strongly. In other words, if you like the smell, it is probably going to work well. You can adapt the recipes for horses to dogs and vice versa, simply adjust the number of drops of oils for each species. Enjoy playing with these recipes, and remember the final choice is always your animal's.

Natural life span

Most of these products will last up to a year stored in a sterilised bottle in the fridge. To extend the shelf life of preservative-free products limit bacterial contamination from the beginning of the creation process till the bottle is finished. To do this you must:

> » Sterilise containers and utensils before use
> » Use latex gloves while making the products
> » Do not put your fingers inside the gel
> » When testing the smell bring a little of the gel to your nose on a spoon, don't put your nose too close to the mixture
> » Use glass or PCR HDPE plastic bottles for storage, with flip-top closures.

Many essential oils control bacterial growth, acting as a preservative. Mixes with high levels of antibacterial oil will last longer than those with minimal essential oil and higher quantities of herbal oil. Finally, you can add a little vitamin E oil, radish root extract or rosemary extract, (available from essential oil suppliers) to increase shelf life by about 50%.

Basic gel recipe

(to make 100 ml of lotion or 250 ml of spray)

Ingredients:

> » Approx 50 ml water based gel (e.g. aloe vera)
> » Up to 10 ml of herbal oil (optional)
> » For horses: a maximum total of 40 drops of essential oil (maximum of 5 different oils per gel)
> » For dogs: a maximum total of 20 drops (maximum 3 different oils)
> » 50-200 ml of distilled water or hydrosol, as per requirement

Procedure

Put the gel in a glass bowl (use utensils made of non-reactive materials such as glass and stainless steel, essential oils can react with plastic and aluminium).

Pour the vegetable oil into a stainless steel measuring spoon and add your chosen essential oils. Mix oils into the gel with a glass stirring rod, or stainless steel whisk.

Slowly whisk in water or hydrosol to thin the gel to your desired consistency.

For a small area on a dog, the gel can be fairly thick, like a rich body lotion. A drop of gel should sit on your hand without spreading. For a large area on a horse, let the gel down with water or hydrosol until it is thin enough to apply with a sponge.

To make a spray, keep adding water or hydrosol until the mix is thin enough to spray.

To make a wash for an after work 'pick-me-up' or as a coat conditioner, add a few squirts of undiluted base gel to a ¼ bucket of water.

Hydrosol gel (100 ml)

Ingredients:

- » 100 ml hydrosol of your choice, or distilled water, or aloe juice
- » 1 teaspoon (Tsp) xanthan or guar gum (available in some food stores and many aromatherapy suppliers)

Procedure:

Use either a hand mixer or blender to make the gel.

First warm the bowl or blender with boiling water, this sterilises the container and makes the hydrosol 'gel' more easily.

Pour hydrosol into the warmed bowl/blender.

Sprinkle the xanthan gum on top of the hydrosol.

Whisk for about 5 minutes or until the xanthan gum has completely dissolved and the gel has thickened

The base gel should be thick enough to hold its shape in your hand without spreading when dropped from a teaspoon. To thin the gel to your desired consistency, stir in more hydrosol or water AFTER you have added any oil or essential oils. Essential oils need to be added into the gel before it is too liquid because they do not dissolve in water and need to be coated with gel to hold them into the solution.

Basic clay recipe (250 ml)

Use wooden or glass utensils.

Ingredients:

» Approx ¼ cup of clay powder (the absorbency varies from clay to clay so you need to experiment with the clays you are using)

» Up to 50 drops of essential oil in total

» Up to 25 ml vegetable oil

» Enough water or hydrosol to bring the clay to the consistency you want

Procedure:

Put the clay in a glass bowl,

Add the essential oils to the vegetable oil,

Pour the oil blend into the clay and mix around.

Slowly add distilled water or hydrosol, mixing with a glass rod until the clay is slightly thinner than you want, as it will thicken more as it stands. Pour it into your storage container before it thickens. If the blend thickens too much, add water and shake well.

RECIPES FOR HORSES

Mud fever (scratches, greasy heel) 250 ml

The clay in this recipe dries out bacteria and the fungi that cause this condition. The clay also protects the leg from excessive moisture. The calendula soothes and heals while the essential oils destroy fungal and bacterial infection. Mud fever heals much better, and does not recur, if you do not wash the leg unless you can completely dry it. Peel off scabs as they come loose, don't force them. Do not clip legs and allow the horse to move as much as possible to encourage circulation. Removing shoes also helps.

Ingredients

» 50 grams bentonite clay

» 30 drops rosalina or manuka essential oil

» 10 drops chamomile, German or yarrow essential oil

» 10 drops myrrh, patchouli or lavender green essential oil

- » 5 drops tea tree, garlic or thyme linalol essential oil
- » 20 ml calendula macerated oil or 10 ml calendula and 10 grams shea butter
- » 100 ml Lavender, witch hazel or cornflower hydrosol
- » 100 ml tea tree or thyme hydrosol

Blend the calendula and shea butter together (warm the shea until it is pourable). Add essential oils to the above, then stir into the clay. Add the hydrosol stirring constantly. Allow to stand for an hour or so, then check the consistency, it should be an easily spreadable, creamy paste. If it is too thin, add more clay; too thick, add more hydrosol.

Sweet itch (250 ml)

In the wild, animals roll in mud and dirt to protect their skin from biting insects, this clay-based recipe protects, heals and strengthens the skin and makes horses less sensitive to bites. Horses that suffer from sweet itch often have an underlying hormonal imbalance or too much heat in the body, so I use essential oils that balance hormones and cool the system.

Ingredients

- » 200 grams kaolin clay
- » 50 ml calendula macerated oil
- » 50 ml neem oil
- » 20 grams shea butter (optional)
- » 150-200 ml hydrosol, geranium, or cistus, or lavender, or witch hazel
- » 20 drops Vitamin E
- » 10 drops chamomile Roman, helichrysum or cistus essential oil
- » 5 drops yarrow essential oil
- » 10 drops vetiver or cedarwood or patchouli
- » 3 drops geranium or ylang ylang or rose or lavender

Combine the vegetable oils and add the essential oils. Stir oils into the clay, then add the hydrosol, stirring constantly. Allow the mixture to stand for an hour or so, then check the consistency. It should be the thickness of good body lotion. If it is too thin, add more clay; too thick, add more hydrosol.

Sarcoids and warts (250 ml)

The less you interfere with sarcoids the better, so resist the temptation to scrub them clean. Apply the clay or gel daily without washing it off in between. As the sarcoid dies, it might break apart and become quite bloody, this is normal and a good sign. Once the sarcoid has a 'neck', you can consult with your vet about tying it off, (wrapping a band to stop the blood flow) as this will hasten its demise. Continue applying oils until the site is completely healed over, so you are sure all rogue cells are destroyed. Generally, it works best to start treating sarcoids with clay and switch to gel to finish the healing after they have dropped off.

Ingredients:

» Either 100 grams green clay or 50 grams bentonite clay or 200 ml gel

» Lavender, or tea tree, or melissa hydrosol, or distilled water

» 40 drops essential of Bergamot or lemon or lentisk

» 20 drops of essential oil of lavender, or tea tree or rosalina

» 10 drops of essential oil of carrot seed, frankincense, seaweed or cedarwood

» If infected you can also consider garlic or thyme

Combine the essential oils. Stir oils into the clay, then add the hydrosol, stirring constantly. Allow the mixture to stand for an hour or so, then check the consistency. It should be the thickness of good body lotion. If it is too thin, add more clay, too thick, add more hydrosol.

Essential oils are very effective against sarcoids, a benign skin tumour of equines, which can grow huge and be difficult to eradicate. Here you see the progress of a sarcoid I treated with a series of clays and gels.

26th October

5 December

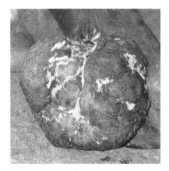
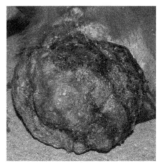

6th December

19th June following year

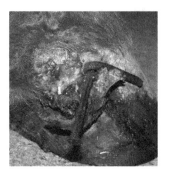
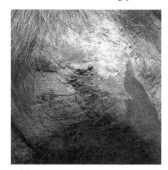

Osteoarthritis (250 ml)

This is a condition where excess bony growth develops around a joint, also known as ringbone and sidebone. The folk cure for this condition was to strap half a lemon to the affected joint, not as silly as it sounds when you consider that lemon essential oil can break down kidney stones.

Ingredients

- » 200 ml Aloe vera, yarrow or peppermint hydrosol gel
- » 20 ml comfrey infused oil
- » 30 drops lemon essential oil
- » 10 drops ginger, peppermint, or rosemary essential oils
- » 5 drops violet leaf absolute or chamomile German, or spearmint essential oil
- » 30 ml distilled water, or hydrosol of witch hazel or peppermint

Add the essential oils to the vegetable oil, stir into the gel. Stir in the hydrosol or water until the gel is the consistency of shampoo.

Sore muscles (100 ml)

Use this for pulled/damaged muscles or just as a liniment after a hard days work. Muscles are connected to the Stomach meridian, so the essential oils that support the stomach also work on the muscles.

Ingredients:

- » 100 ml aloe vera gel or peppermint, rosemary or thyme hydrosol gel
- » 10 drops essential oil of Plai, or ginger, or thyme

» 10 drops essential oil of lemongrass, or spearmint, or rosemary, or basil

» 5 drops essential oil of nutmeg, or marjoram, or clary sage

Add the essential oils to the gel. Stir or shake well.

Tendons and ligaments (100 ml)

Just as the Stomach meridian relates to muscles, Liver meridian supports healthy tendons and ligaments. If your horse suffers from frequent tendon problems, I suggest you give him herbs and essential oils to cleanse his liver.

Ingredients:

» 85 ml aloe vera gel, or peppermint, yarrow, rosemary or juniper berry hydrosol gel

» 15 ml comfrey infused oil

» 10 drops roman chamomile, blue chamomile, yarrow essential oil

» 10 drops juniper berry, or seaweed, or plai

» 5 drops helichrysum

Add the essential oils to the vegetable oil, stir into the gel.

Hoof gel (250 ml)

In the wild, horses moisturise their feet daily as they stand in the water when they drink. This gel replicates the 'feet in water' moisturising method, without oily additions that can actually soften feet too much, or prevent them 'breathing'.

Ingredients:

» 125 ml thyme or tea tree hydrosol, or 100 ml aloe vera gel

» Essential oils:

  » 20 drops carrot seed

  » 10 drops Rosemary, or thyme, or eucalyptus

  » 5 drops or vetiver, or patchouli

  » 5 drops seaweed absolute, or 5 ml seaweed extract

  » Add 125 ml (or as needed) of carrot seed, cornflower, chamomile, witch hazel or lavender hydrosol (or a combination)

Add the essential oils to the vegetable oil, stir into the gel. Stir in the hydrosol or water until the gel is the consistency of shampoo.

Thrush or other hoof infections, including white line disease (250 ml)

Make a thick clay that you can pack into the hoof. This protects the foot from wetness, draws out infection, dries out fungi and holds the anti-bacterial and anti-fungal essential oils in place. Be careful not to get this mix on healthy skin as it is quite harsh and prolonged contact could cause discomfort. Reapply daily.

Ingredients:

- » 100-150 grams of green clay
- » 200 ml thyme, or tea tree, hydrosol
- » Essential oils:
- » 10 drops garlic, or lentisk, or tea tree, or thyme,
- » 20 drops eucalyptus, or rosemary, or manuka, lavender green. You could also divide the drops between two of these
- » 2 drops seaweed absolute (optional)

Combine the essential oils and clay, add hydrosol and stir or shake well, the final clay should be thick as cookie dough. Pack into a well-cleaned hoof and use a hard brush to work well into cracks. For persistent deep cracks you can mix essential oils in 50% apple cider vinegar 50% hydrosol and inject with a small syringe

Sunburn

White-nosed horses or dogs can be prone to sunburn. This gel will help heal painful condition quickly and should be applied in the evening. The clay sunscreen protects from the sun's rays, soothes the skin and repairs damaged cells, making the skin stronger and less sensitive. Apply a light layer every morning, or when the sun is strong.

After sun gel – 100 ml

- » 100 ml aloe vera gel or lavender hydrosol gel
- » 5 ml St John's wort oil
- » 5 drops lavender essential oil
- » 5 drops rosalina (optional)

Add the essential oils to the vegetable oil, stir into the gel. Stir in the hydrosol or water until the gel is the consistency of shampoo.

Clay sunscreen – 250 ml

- » 15 grams of shea butter,
- » 10 ml of sesame oil
- » 10 drops lavender essential oil
- » ¼ cup kaolin clay
- » 200 ml lavender, cornflower or witch hazel hydrosol.

Gently heat the butter in a double boiler till it is soft enough to blend with the oil, add essential oil, stir in clay, slowly add hydrosol until its a loose lotion.

Wound ointment (100 ml)

You could use clay instead of gel for this recipe if you want to have more of a protective or drawing effect.

Ingredients:

- » 90 ml aloe gel or tea tree or lavender or cistus hydrosol gel
- » 10 ml calendula and/or comfrey infused oil
- » Essential oils:
- » 10 drops tea tree or rosalina or manuka
- » 10 drops lavender or cistus
- » 5 drops yarrow or chamomile German, or helichrysum

Add the essential oils to the vegetable oil, stir into the gel. Stir in the hydrosol or water until the gel is the consistency shampoo.

Fly spray concentrate (500 ml makes 5 litres of spray)

You can be creative in combining the oils you use for fly spray, play around till you find what works for you and your horse. The actual insecticidal ingredient is neem oil. I make up a concentrate and then dilute my daily requirement with hydrosol or distilled water (depending how bad the flies are), right in the fly sprayer, or in a bucket of water to sponge on.

Ingredients:

- » 125 ml aloe vera gel or eucalyptus, lemongrass, lavender or peppermint hydrosol gel
- » 100-200 ml neem oil

» 40 drops essential oil

» Combine all the ingredients then add Hydrosol to make up to 500 ml

Many essential oils are deterrent to bugs, these are some of the top ones, but don't let the list restrict you:

» Cedarwood, eucalyptus (especially citriodora), lavender, lemongrass, garlic, geranium, marjoram, peppermint, thyme, vetiver, patchouli, ylang ylang.

To make the spray, add the concentrate to a spray bottle, add water or hydrosol and 10 ml of apple cider vinegar per litre of liquid and shake vigorously. For example, for a standard 500 ml spray bottle, add 50 ml of concentrate, 5 ml of apple cider vinegar and 455 ml of liquid. If your bugs are really bad you can make the spray stronger by using more concentrate.

RECIPES FOR DOGS

I use topical applications less on dogs less than I do on horses, simply because they do not need as much of them. Any of the recipes for horses could also be adapted for dogs by using less essential oils. I have found that dogs often prefer not to have essential oils applied topically and prefer recipes made with hydrosols. You can replace any of the essential oils mentioned with its hydrosol if that is the case for your dog. Below are recipes that are for specifically 'doggy' problems.

Arthritis gel (100 ml)

Apply to affected joints on days that your dog looks more stiff or sore. You can also put a few drops of juniper berry, yarrow or ginger hydrosol in a saucer of water for them to drink when they like.

Ingredients

» 50 ml aloe vera gel, or make a gel from ginger, yarrow or juniper berry hydrosol

» Essential oils:

  » 3 drops ginger

  » 3 drops lavender or violet leaf absolute

  » 5 drops yarrow or German chamomile

  » 5 drops juniper berry, cedarwood or cypress

  » 10 ml St John's wort infused oil or hemp seed oil (optional)

Add essential oils to the infused oil and then stir into the gel. If you don't use infused oil, stir the essential oils straight into the gel. Slowly stir in up to 50 ml of one of the hydrosols listed above until you reach the required consistency.

Itchy skin (100 ml)

Often the cause of itchy skin is diet: remove wheat, soy and other known allergens from a dogs diet, preferably feed fresh meat or moist food, not dried food. Stress can also cause itching, as can pain.

Ingredients

- » 50 ml aloe vera gel, or gel of witch hazel, lavender, chamomile, cistus
- » 10 ml calendula infused oil
- » 5 drops lavender essential oil
- » 5 drops, Roman or German chamomile, or yarrow, or helichrysum
- » 3 drops vetiver, or myrhh, or patchouli

Add essential oils to the infused oil, and then stir into the gel. If you don't use infused oil, stir the essential oils straight into the gel. Slowly stir in up to 50 ml of the hydrosols until you reach the required consistency.

Wet excema (100 ml)

Before application, clean and dry affected area thoroughly and clip back hair. Feed your dog cooling or neutral food as described in Chapter 6, The Stress Factor. If your dog doesnt like the aromatics you can just sprinkle dry clay on the area.

Ingredients:

- » 2 teaspoons bentonite clay
- » 10 ml calendula infused oil (optional but highly recommended)
- » Essential oils:
  - » 5 drops lavender or lavender green
  - » 5 drops myrrh, or patchouli
  - » 50 ml tea tree or cistus hydrosol
  - » 50 ml distilled water.

Add essential oils to the infused oil and then stir into the clay. Add the hydrosol to the clay, stir or shake vigorously then allow it to sit for two to 12 hours stirring occasionally until the clay is fully absorbed.

Fungal infection (100 ml)

Fungi thrive on damp, so deprive them of the moist conditions they love and they can't survive. A major cause of internal Damp is a cereal-based diet, feed a slightly warm meat-based diet.

Ingredients:

- » 2 tablespoons green clay
- » 5 ml calendula infused oil (optional)
- » Essential oils:
    - » 5 drops roman or chamomile (German)
    - » 2 drops tea tree, rosalina, or manuka
    - » 1 drop patchouli, frankincense or myrrh
    - » 100 ml lavender or thyme hydrosol

Flea and tick repellent (100 ml)

Rub a small amount of this gel into the animal's coat, paying special attention to ears, belly and 'armpits'. You can also make this gel thin enough to use as a spray if you prefer by using only 20 ml of gel to start with.

- » 50 ml aloe vera gel, or gel from tea tree, lavender or lemongrass hydrosol
- » 10 ml neem oil
- » 50 ml geranium, eucalyptus or peppermint hydrosol (or what you've used above),
- » Essential oils:
    - » 5 drops cedarwood, cypress or juniper berry
    - » 4 drops lavender, lemongrass, or geranium
    - » 1 drops patchouli, marjoram, or ylang ylang

Add essential oils to the infused oil and then stir into the gel. If you don't use infused oil, stir the essential oils straight into the gel. Slowly stir in up to 50 ml of hydrosol to required consistency.

Ear wash (10 ml)

This is a pleasant way to wash out your dogs ears and keep on top of the black gunk. Be aware that black gunk and fungal ear infections are often a symptom of underlying immune weakness or a poor diet, feed a grain free diet and reduce stress to strengthen immune function. Don't use essential oil inside the ear.

» 5 ml thyme or tea tree hydrosol (antibacterial)

» 2.5 ml Lavender or chamomile hydrosol (soothing)

» 2.5 ml yarrow or myrrh hydrosol

» 1 ml calendula macerated or olive oil

Bad breath (30 ml)

I am often asked which essential oils are good against bad breath. My standard answer is bad breath comes from a bad diet. Bad breath will disappear if you give your dog or cat fresh meat and meaty bones. However, if your dog has gingivitis try:

» 10 ml thyme or tea tree hydrosol

» 15 ml Myrrh or lentisk hydrosol

» 10-15 ml aloe vera gel

Mix the myrrh/lentisk with the aloe gel, then add thyme/tea tree hydrosol and stir well. You should have a thin paste that you can smear on your finger and rub onto your dogs gums. Do this as long as your dog allows it. If you can't rub the mix on your dog's gums, mix the solution in about 100 ml of water and leave it down for your dog to drink if he wishes. You can also make a clay version of this, which some dogs prefer, just replace the aloe gel with green or bentonite clay.

Deodorant

I am often asked for 'dog perfume' - no, not a fragrance to make you smell like a dog, (although your furry friend would probably prefer that), something to make dogs smell more like us. If your dog doesn't smell good, feed it better food! A healthy dog smells good. If you must try to make a dog smell 'un-doggy' you can use hydrosols as a rinse or spray, but let your dog choose her own scent.

RECIPES FOR CATS

Cats are sensitive to essential oils and you should never apply them topically. However, if you must, you can use hydrosols for flea repellent or wound cleaning. You can make a gel to rub in, or spray hydrosol directly onto the cat's fur. As most cats do not enjoy this very much, I only do it when there is a real need.

My favourite natural flea control for cats (I also use it on dogs) is diatomaceous earth. This is a naturally occurring powder made of fossilised remains of microscopic one-celled plants (phytoplankton) called diatoms that lived in the oceans and lakes that once covered the western part of the US and other parts of the world. These deposits are mined from underwater beds or from ancient dried lake bottoms. It is a very fine powder that physically damages the exo-skeleton of insects that move through it, causing them to die. It is important to use food grade diatomaceous earth. Avoid breathing it in when dusting, but apart from that it is non-toxic and effective.

Cat's flea and tick repellent (100 ml) also good for puppies

- » 15 ml aloe gel
- » 5 ml neem oil
- » 40 ml hydrosol of geranium, or lavender, or lemongrass, or frankincense, or rosemary, or a combination of two of them
- » 40 ml distilled water

Add the neem oil to the aloe gel and mix well, slowly add the hydrosols your cat selected and the water. Rub a small amount through your cats coat, against the lie of the fur, paying particular attention to the flea pathways: between the back legs, around the tail and ears and ruff of the neck, and along the spine.

Flea repellent 2

This works well for dogs as well, and I even use a version of it on my horses to prevent ticks.

- » 1cup Diatomaceous earth
- » ½ cup neem leaf powder
- » ¼ cup white clay

Mix together gently and avoid breathing in the dust. Put into a plastic squeezy buttle with a flip top lid. To apply brush fur backwards at the ruff of the neck and squeeze powder onto the skin, working it in gently with your fingers. I also apply to armpits and tummy. It is ok for them to lick the powder.

Wounds

You can wash cat wounds with hydrosols: cistus yarrow, lavender, witch hazel, tea tree (dilute 50%) or thyme (dilute 75%) with distilled water or add to aloe vera gel.

Cat bite clay

This is one instance where topical application can be helpful as the clay draws out any toxins injected with the cat's bite and helps the wound heal without infection. Be warned, if an abscess is already forming the wound may look worse before it looks better as it will open up before it closes. The wound should look significantly better within eight hours of application, if your cat is extremely subdued or has a raised temperature he needs veterinary attention.

Ingredients:
- » Thyme or tea tree hydrosol
- » Distilled Water
- » green clay

Make a thick paste from green clay using 50% thyme and 50% distilled water. Smother the wound with the clay and stop the cat licking it off for at least 10 minutes if you can. Clean with soapy or salty water and re-apply daily until the wound looks clean and is healing well (usually a day or two), or until your cat struggles and does not want it applied. You can then offer to dab the wound with lavender hydrosol. Even if your cat is uncooperative (let's be realistic here) and you manage only one application of clay and don't wash it off, the wound is much more likely to heal quickly and cleanly.

Gingivitis drops

Cats and dogs often suffer from poor dental health, this is mostly because they do not have access to fresh meaty bones, which clean and stimulate a carnivore's gums. The first step for any dog or cat with yucky teeth or gums is to give them a bone! Dogs like large meaty bones. The perfect tooth brush for a cat is a raw chicken neck. Along with this, you can use hydrosols and squirt them into your cat's mouth with an eye dropper if he will allow it, or put them in a saucer for him to self-medicate. You can also make them into a gel and rub a little into your cat's gums.

- » 10 ml lentisk hydrosol
- » 5 drops myrrh hydrosol
- » 10 ml distilled water

Mix well and store in dropper bottle.

I was once adopted by a five-week-old kitten who lived in a garbage skip on Katz street. He was infested with ear mites, had lost one eye to infection and his gums were infected. To be honest he stank. The vet told me he would need to clean the gums under anaesthetic once the kitten was healthy enough. Meanwhile I washed Mr Katz' ears out daily (see dog recipes for my ear wash) and gave him raw chicken neck twice a day. I also washed his mouth with the gingivitis drops once a day. Within days his ears were mite free and his gums were starting to look normal. When I took him in for a check up a month later his adult teeth had all come through and were bright white in healthy pink gums, much to the vet's surprise.

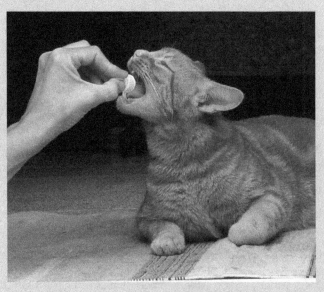

"We live longer than our forefathers; but we suffer more from a thousand artificial anxieties and cares. They fatigued only the muscles, we exhaust the finer strength of the nerves."

- Edward George Bulwer-Lytton

CHAPTER 6

———

THE STRESS FACTOR

I can't leave you without a few words on stress as it is such an integral part of how I approach animal health.

When I first started working with essential oils I found that in some cases my animal clients improved a certain amount, but didn't heal completely. A few cases didn't lose interest in the oils, others showed no interest in the oils at all. In each of these situations the problem cleared up completely once I had identified and removed the source of stress. Often this was as simple as giving oils to other pack members as well, changing the diet, or moving a cat's litter box.

Aromatic extracts reduce stress and can help animals cope with living in a stressful environment, but for true health we must reduce environmental stress where possible. By understanding our animals' natural needs, we can reduce stress in their lives and help them stay healthy. The following chapter helps you understand and recognise stress, how to minimise stress in your animals' lives and suggests essential oils/hydrosols for specific stress-related problems.

WHAT IS STRESS?

The word 'stress' is so widely used in our culture today that the true meaning of the word has been obscured. We claim to 'get stressed' by a heavy workload, or family strife, or by little things like deciding what to wear, or waiting in lines in the supermarket. But what is stress actually? And is it always a bad thing?

Simply put, stress is a physiological response to anything that an animal perceives as threatening to its well-being; the threat could be an angry bear or a lack of food, indigestion or injury.

Most domesticated animals are subjected to stress of one kind or another in the course of their daily life. Even if nothing traumatic has ever happened to them, we have taken the animal out of the environment where it evolved, feed it food it was not designed to eat, and deprive it of some of its basic physiological requirements, such as freedom of movement.

STRESS IS NATURAL

Every animal is hard-wired to deal with a certain amount of acute stress, especially prey animals, who must remain alert if they are to survive. The stress response is a mechanism essential for survival, a sudden bio-chemical jolt that puts all systems on alert, ready to either flee or fight; without it we would not survive.

Functions not essential to surviving the immediate problem are shut down or reduced. Once the animal has acted to remove the danger, a second release of hormones returns the body to a relaxed and balanced state. The system works well as long as an animal can remove the stress. But if the stress is always present the body never normalises. This leads to distress and a wide variety of problems such as itchy skin, digestive upsets and maladaptive behaviours.

How the stress response affects the body	
Increased activity	Suppressed activity
Increased respiration, Rapid shallow breathing	Constriction of most blood vessels
Dilated blood vessels in heart & limb muscles	Decreased blood clotting time
Increased skeletal muscle strength	Reduced intestinal movement
Increased heart rate	Inhibited secretions e.g. tears, digestive juices
Increased sugar and fat levels in the blood	Bladder relaxes
Dilated pupils	Inhibited erection or vaginal lubrication
Increased perspiration	Suppressed immune function
Increased mental activity	
More white blood cells at skin surface	

IDENTIFYING STRESS

Some animals develop behaviours easily recognisable as a stress response such as:

Excess barking

Stereo-typical behaviours

Box-walking

Fur or feather plucking

Tail chasing

Marking and urinating

However, many signs of stress can be easily overlooked:

Bumping into you, or tripping you up	Guarding food or people
Scratching or rubbing	Inability to play
Controlling movement of others	Hiding
Lack of eye contact	Aggression
Lack of adaptability	Lack of concentration

When stress manifests in the body the skin is often the first place to suffer, e.g:

Increased sensitivity to fleas/flies	Excessive scratching or rubbing
Slow healing wounds	Chronic infections
Poor quality coat or hooves	Allergic reactivity
Hotspots	

Other common stress-related illnesses include:

Colic	Chronic coughs and colds
Irritable bowel syndrome	Weight loss or chronically underweight
Muscle tightness	Frequent injury
'Is he-isn't he?' lameness	Auto-immune disease

Some behaviours, particularly excess licking or rubbing, can be a sign of either mental stress or pain. Dogs with 'hot-spots' who lick obsessively often have underlying pain, although this condition is frequently attributed to mental stress. Animals will often lick and rub at acupuncture points along the meridians in an attempt to stimulate or calm them. Any physical pain is likely to cause licking, scratching or rubbing.

I consider any illness or behaviour that is abnormal for that particular animal as early warning that the body/mind system is stressed. An alert animal guardian will notice any change in behaviour, attitude, movement, or smell, find the cause and remove the stressor before it can develop into a more serious problem.

THE STRESS BANK

It is impossible and undesirable to keep our animals 100% stress free, a small amount of stress from time to time helps animals learn how to respond to stressors appropriately. Our responsibility as animal guardians is to prevent them from suffering from stress.

An animal in good health, mentally and physically, will have no problem dealing with the stresses of life and will be less affected when faced with a stressor, such as moving house, changing hands, exposure to a virus, or fireworks. An animal who is already stressed on a daily basis is more likely to become ill when exposed to a virus, or moving house. Or may suddenly become noise phobic after one loud crash.

Animals cope with stress more or less efficiently depending on genetics, early life experience and how you take care of them. However, even if they have effective coping mechanisms and a supportive environment, any on-going stress will take its toll on the body eventually.

Think of it as banking - we all come into life with a stress allowance that we draw upon when times get rough, but if we are constantly making withdrawals (chronic stress) without making a deposit (removing stressors) we will end up in debt. You can be in debt for a short time, especially if your credit has always been good, but if you keep drawing on your allowance you will end up bankrupt.

So, for every withdrawal you must make a deposit: if you ride your horse (withdrawal), make sure his saddle fits, that you are straight and balanced, that he is doing work that he enjoys (minimising stress), and make sure he has enough time for free movement, hanging out with his friends, and rolling so he can work the kinks out of his body (deposit). Otherwise your horse is likely to become 'snappy' or depressed as he expresses his discomfort (stress), leading to lameness (debt) if you do not heed the early signs.

If you have more than two cats (a stressor for many cats), make sure that everyone has their own litter tray, a safe place of their own, and safe passage from area to area (deposit), otherwise you are likely to have problems with inappropriate spraying and cat-to-cat aggression (debt). If you have a dog that eats only commercial dried food (withdrawal) give her fresh bones sometimes and a chance to detox by eating grasses or clay/mud (deposit), otherwise she can develop itchy skin, bad breath and infected gums (debt).

BALANCING THE BANK

Following are some common causes of stress in a domestic environment, actions you can take to reduce or eradicate these stressors, and essential oils that can help. This list will also help you to look around your environment and see it through your animal's eyes, maybe you can find even more ways to enrich your friend's life.

Danger

Domestic situations that can make an animal feel threatened include: living with unknown or unfriendly 'others', lack of respect from people, angry body language.

Solution: Don't force animals that threaten each other to live close to each other; treat animals with respect and kindness; keep your body language non-threatening; build trust with your animals so they feel safe.

Essential oil/hydrosol: Any calming oil, especially frankincense, clary sage, jasmine.

Illness

Illness is a stress as well as an outcome of stress as it strains physical resources and makes an animal feel vulnerable. In the wild, animals often hide away until they are well.

Solution: Reduce all other stressors when an animal is ill; provide a safe quiet environment; use essential oils to stimulate immune system and reduce stress.

Essential oil/hydrosol: Almost all essential oils support immune function. Key immune stimulants are lemon, angelica root, ravensara, vetiver.

Accident

Accidents trigger a massive stress response. Even minor accidents interfere with the body's 'electric circuits' (flow of energy) and can cause imbalances that lead to physical and behavioural problems. Medical procedures and aftercare also cause physical and mental stress.

Solution: Reset the 'electric circuits' using essential oils, acupuncture/pressure, or kinesiology; detox the body with essential oils, herbs, clay.

Essential oil/hydrosol: Yarrow, helichrysum, juniper berry, seaweed, carrot seed.

Chronic Pain

Many displays of bad temper or poor condition in horses arise from underlying pain. Dogs and cats will often have a change of temperament when in pain and this is sometimes the only sign you will see.

Solution: Allow horses to roll and buck freely to release stiffness; take shoes off; check saddle fit; make sure you are balanced and supple when riding; give dogs time to warm up and warm down before exertion; reduce stress so muscles can relax; provide hands-on healing, cranio-sacral, Bowen technique, massage.

Essential oil/hydrosol: Marjoram, yarrow, ginger, peppermint, plai.

Vaccination

Latest research reveals that we are over-vaccinating. Animals, like humans, need an initial series of vaccinations for most of the major diseases, such as rabies and parvo-virus, which will give life-long immunity. Vaccinating can cause cancer at the site of injection for cats and rabies vaccinosis in dogs and challenges the immune system.

Solution: Examine your vaccination programme, balance the likelihood of exposure to disease, against the risk of immune stress; ask your vet to do blood titers to test for immunity; use homeopathic nosodes; where annual vaccination is a legal requirement, use homeopathic remedies or essential oils to neutralise the side effects and detox.

Essential oil/hydrosol: Carrot seed, juniper berry, grapefruit.

Synthetic chemicals

A healthy, stress-free animal may deal with chemical exposure, but it can be the feather that tips the balance for others. Common irritants for dogs and cats are carpet cleaners and plug-in air fresheners.

Solution: Use bio-friendly cleaning products; feed organic foods where practical; make sure your pets can get away from air-fresheners whether they are natural or synthetic.

Pest control

Spot-ons, flea collars and fly sprays are supposed to be safe for pets and humans, 'relatively safe' would be more accurate. It is sensible to question your need for chemical intervention and try to control fleas/flies naturally if possible.

Solution: Balance the risk of exposure against the risk of stress (an indoor cat has little need for pest control, whereas dogs in areas of tick-borne disease do need); use natural bug control, neem-based products are best. Feed a natural diet to support natural bug-repellency; reduce stress.

Essential oil/hydrosol: Many essential oils are insect repellent, let your animal choose. Use neem as base oil, eucalyptus, lavender, patchouli, cedarwood, lemongrass.

Worming

Wormers also take a toll on the body's detoxification system. Animals (including humans) can live quite happily with a low level of worms. Research has linked an increase in asthma and allergic responses to an absence of parasitic worms.

Solution: Do faecal worm count regularly, only worm when needed. Clear droppings in horse pasture; provide access to vermifuge herbs and clay; use natural wormers; provide coarse grasses for dogs and cats to self worm.

Essential oils/hydrosols: Bergamot, carrot seed, thyme.

Processed food

Processed food and diets high in sugars (molasses, 'industrial' hay & grass), indigestible protein (soy, maize) and poor quality ingredients are a leading cause of skin, behaviour and musculo-skeletal problems.

Solution: Feed a species-specific diet, meat-based for dogs and cats, forage for horses, avoid soy, wheat and maize, preservatives, colourings and sugars. Do not overfeed.

Weaning

Animals in the wild only suffer sudden weaning if the mother dies or disappears, leaving the youngster to fend for itself, without much chance of survival. Many behaviour problems, fears and insecurities arise from weaning too early; it also means youngsters don't learn social skills.

Solution: Leave weaning to the mother if you can; horses, wean into a herd with mixed ages, so they have guidance and security, from elders; make sure dogs and cats are not left alone until mature enough to deal with it; reduce all other stressors.

Essential oils/hydrosols: Neroli, violet leaf absolute, chamomile Roman, sweet orange.

Confinement

Cats need a large 'personal space' so being confined to a house can be stressful, especially for males. The homeostasis of a horse is based on free movement, confinement puts stress on the whole system. Most dogs are happy to lie around doing nothing 'in the den' but need regular exercise and social interaction.

Solution: Provide as much space as possible for your horses to roam; if confinement is necessary for healing an injury, offer essential oils; give cats room to hide; dogs need company.

Essential oils/hydrosols: Frankincense, lentisk, peppermint, rosemary, eucalyptus.

Isolation

Solitary confinement is one of the worst punishments for any social animal. To flourish, all animals need the touch and smell of their own species, especially herd animals. They also need mental and physical stimulation.

Solution: Horses: provide company, preferably a 'family' herd of mixed ages and sexes. Dogs: provide free association with their own species; do not leave them home alone. Cats: provide toys to play with; allow access to the outside, even if it is only a window ledge.

Overcrowding

Every animal needs a certain amount of 'personal space' to feel comfortable. Animals who live in groups need to be able to distance themselves from each other to signal submission and reduce tensions. Overcrowding increases aggression and competition for food.

Solution: Do not overcrowd! As a minimum requirement, each horse should be able to stand in an imaginary circle with a radius of two horse lengths without touching another horse's circle; each dog in the house should have its own bed; cats should each have a distinct territory and not have to share litter trays.

Changes in routine or environment

Loss of control of one's own environment is a major stress. Animals who are dependent on others to provide their needs can become very distressed when their routine changes.

Solution: Keep your routine flexible, or change routines slowly, reduce all other stresses so unexpected changes in routine are not such a big deal.

Essential oil/hydrosol: Cedarwood, cypress, geranium, violet leaf absolute.

Boredom

In a natural environment the daily search for food, water and shelter, plus the social inter-action of a group of animals, provides all the mental, physical and emotional interaction an animal needs; a domestic environment often does not. Repetitive work can also be stressful.

Solution: Turn your horse out with a herd; let your dog play with other dogs; play with your animal, teach him tricks (yes even cats!); avoid repetition when training.

Essential oil/hydrosol: Peppermint, rosemary, lemon.

Over stimulation

Kennels, stable yards, loud music, busy families, high energy training, can all over-stimulate. Animals need a safe place to rest properly and enough time between adrenalin bursts for the relaxation response to be effective.

Solution: Turn down loud radios in stable yards, or tune them to soothing music; make sure dogs and cats have a safe place to retreat from hustle-bustle; reward calm behaviour with at-tention, ignore excitement.

Essential oil/hydrosol: Many essential oils are relaxing or sedative, e.g. Roman chamomile, clary sage, frankincense, lavender, valerian, ylang ylang.

THE HUMAN AS STRESSOR

Finally, one of the most common causes of stress for animals is humans. The good thing about this is, that if we are the cause, we can also be the solution: it is entirely in our hands.

You could say that humans are the only source of chronic stress for domestic animals, after all if it weren't for us they would be living free and wild. But then, the natural lifestyle is not necessarily stress-free either.

I do not advocate turning all our animals loose, I tried it once and my horses were all back in the corral as fast as they could gallop! For better or worse we are their caretakers, our respon-sibility is to be a good guardian and an attentive student. What animals ask from us is that we respect them as individuals, provide them with a home that fulfils their inherent needs, and learn the lessons they offer us every day.

Most people who keep animals love them and want to care for them in the best way possible, but many accepted animal husbandry practices – ways we have been taught are 'right' – are stressors in themselves. Concerned pet owners will seek to educate themselves about what motivates an animal and how we can best fulfil their physiological and psychological needs. This often means letting go of ingrained ideas, not always easy for humans to do.

Training methods can be a stressor for dogs and horses. All animals learn naturally through play and listen to the leader out of desire and respect; any training method that does not work on these principles is stressful. Humans are goal-orientated creatures, always in a hurry to 'get there', so we tend to over-train, never allowing time for the brain to absorb what it has learned, and forgetting to reward each tiny step in the right direction.

Humans, naturally, see the world from a human-centric perspective and project human motives and desires onto their pets. Your dog rubs against you and you think it wants love, or to say it loves you, when actually it is trying to say 'I am top dog around here, pet me when I command'. Emotional transference and lack of understanding of body language creates a large percentage of the problems that I see on a daily basis, but they are mostly easily resolved with a little education. One of the main ways to reduce stress is by understanding yourself better. Explore your motives, desires and emotions and what you are saying with your body. This brings clearer communication with your animals and a happier, healthier life for all.

Remember, you don't have to remove every stress from your animal's life, so don't panic if your lifestyle does not allow you to provide all conditions - I certainly don't want you to 'stress' about it! Even if you can't provide your horses 400 acres of wilderness or your dog a pack of friends to roam with, just do what your circumstances allow. Simply listening to your pet's needs will reduce stress and put lots of credit in the bank.

FEEDING FOR HEALTH

What we eat affects both body and mind and an unsuitable diet is one of the major causes of physical and mental stress for animals. Diet is also an easy place for animal guardians to start making a positive impact on the stress balance. Here is a little background on why I make this claim and simple ways you can feed for health.

The Great Pet Food Whitewash!

In the last decades nutrition has become a science, food has been broken down and analysed, and scientists have told us exactly how much our animals need to eat of each nutrient. On paper the numbers all add up. Theoretically our pets should be feeling healthier. Hhowever, an alarming number of animals suffer from food sensitivities, digestive problems, obesity, hyperactivity, bad breath and excessive shedding.

In the not so distant past, dogs ate man's left-overs, horses ate grass, hay and whole oats, and cats ate mice! They survived on this diet for centuries, yet experts have convinced us that we cannot feed our animals anything that is not formulated by a nutritionist.

Modern feeding practices for most domestic animals have developed for ease of use and profitability. Most commercially produced animal food is based on ingredients that would not normally be part of that species' diet, and is therefore indigestible. Dogs and cats are fed scraps left by meat processors as unfit for human consumption. These scraps are ground, heated and mixed with cereals and soybeans (vegetable protein), coloured to make them appealing to the human eye, sprayed with flavourings to make them palatable, and then preserved so they can sit in a bag for a year.

Nowadays there is a growing number among those caring for horses, who put a lot of time and effort into providing their horses an "as natural" life style. Despite this, the majority of captive horses are fed measured meals at set times of day. Not only are these meals always the same, they are often high in cereals and sugars, but low in carbohydrates, and again, so highly processed that most of the naturally occurring nutrients have been destroyed. Further nutrients are destroyed as the feed sits in bags for months on end.

Feed the individual

So what should we do? With a little understanding of nutritional requirements and some common sense, all animal guardians can feed their animals a convenient and natural diet - without breaking the bank (stress or piggy). Through my practice with animals and by observing the animals that live with me, I have developed a view of nutrition that:

>> Considers the individual

>> Provides a species specific diet as much as is practically possible

>> Uses the Chinese medical view of balanced feeding for health.

Species-specific diet

Each species has evolved over hundreds of thousands of years to eat certain foods, their digestive system, bone structure and mentality is keyed to this end. Dogs are probably the most adaptive of our common pets, having lived in our houses for so long and eaten our scraps for millennia. But, just as our modern diet has become more processed and packaged for convenience, so has our canine friends' diet. With the same disastrous results.

Providing a diet as close as conveniently possible to natural is an obvious and simple choice. Here are brief descriptions of the natural diet of our three most common companions, and ways you can mimic that in a domestic envrionment. The the same principles apply to all creatures, if you understand their natural diet. I recommend you read further on this subject, particularly if you are about to take up raw feeding. See the bibliography.

NATURAL DIET OF THE EQUID

Horses eat all day long so their stomach is never empty and their day is filled with the search for food. Food sources change through the seasons. In the spring, there is an abundance of flowers and grasses, rich in sugars and complex carbohydrates but also rich in herbs that cleanse the blood and stimulate the liver. They get fat and glossy. In summer, when the days are long, the grass is less rich, but a certain amount of ripe grain is available on the stalk. They will lose some weight, but will not have to cover as much ground to find their food, and they are likely to eat clay or dirt to counteract the high tannin content of summer plants. As autumn arrives, horses browse leaves, berries, twigs and other fibre-rich foods to gain weight before winter's cold. In winter, they will eat whatever they find, dried grass stalks with grain, branches, roots, dried fruit, pine needles and nuts. They will lose weight and have to travel far to find enough to eat.

Feeding Horses

Good quality forage (grass, hay, chaff etc.) should always be the basis of any equine diet. This will provide the energy needs of most horses working today. There are even endurance horses competing successfully who eat an entirely forage-based diet, (pelleted alfalfa and other grasses, along with un-molassed sugar beet). If fast burning energy is required (for instance, for an older horse or a race horse), add soaked whole oats and a feed balancer.

You can replicate nature's variety by offering fresh or dried herbs; favourites are rosehips, calendula, devil's claw, yarrow, burdock root, plantain and dandelion, but look around you and see what is in season. You can also add fresh fruit and vegetables, soaked seaweed, a cup full of green clay in a bucket of water, and branches of non-poisonous trees. Branches are particularly appreciated in autumn.

NATURAL DIET OF THE CANINE

Dogs have evolved over thousands of years to eat raw meat and bones. Logically, this must be the food best suited to them. There is even an argument that dogs from different geographical areas of the world have evolved to eat variations on this basic wild diet, so different breeds might be more suited to one protein source e.g. collies to lamb, huskies to fish.

Dogs eat the whole carcass including fur, neural tissue and gut contents, starting with the viscera (liver, stomach etc.), including the gut content (semi-digested grass, cereal and vegetable matter), then move onto muscle and other tissues. Finally they are left with bones to chew, which cleans their teeth. The action of tearing and ripping at the carcass works their teeth, ripping up the skin acts like dental floss, all of this is essential for healthy gums and teeth. As hunters, canids expend a great deal of energy catching their food and are not always successful, in which case they might go hungry for a day. Fasting once in a while is good for a dog's digestion, as is exercising before a meal.

NATURAL DIET OF THE FELINE

Cats are one of the planet's most efficient predators and as such their digestive systems are not adapted to synthesise nutrients from vegetable matter. They are obliagate carnivores, meat should constitute at least 80% of their diet. Cats usually consume small prey whole, larger prey is often only partially eaten, leaving digestive tract, skin, hair, larger bones, or feathers. Larger prey may be eaten over several days, although cats seldom take carrion.

The domestic cat's main prey is small mammals such as rodents and rabbits, birds, reptiles and insects. Due to the relatively small size of their prey, small cats must hunt several times a day to fulfil their nutritional needs, and they are always on the lookout for

My 7 Principles of Feeding for Health

Principle	Which means...
Species specific	Each species has evolved over millennia to eat in a way that best suits its physical needs, so work with nature and provide the appropriate diet.
Individual	Each individual within a species has specific requirements, you cannot feed every animal in the same way.
Climate	One of the main considerations for the individual is its Climate, as seen by the Chinese medical system, this relates to its Element.
Variety	Naturally speaking, diet changes according to availability and season. Eating one ingredient all the time can cause sensitisation, plus it reduces the range of available nutrients.
Choice	Provide animals the opportunity to choose what they need for a balanced diet; do not force them to eat things they do not want.
Quality	Food should always be fresh and clean and the highest quality available.
Easy	Design a diet that is easy for you to provide, do not cause yourself stress by thinking you must only feed one way, remember the stress bank and do what you can.

their next meal. Cats do not have an effective hunger 'shut off' mechanism. Cats are designed to receive 80% of their liquid requirements from their prey.

Feeding canines and felines

The single most important thing in feeding cats and dogs is to provide meat as the protein. This may seem obvious, but often the protein in pet food is derived from vegetables, such as soya. Ideally, dogs and cats will eat raw meat as the basis of their diet. Dogs also need a small amount of partly processed (liquidised or lightly steamed) vegetables, unless they have free access to grasses and herbivore droppings. To get all the nutrients they require they must eat muscle meat, organ meat and bones.

In my experience, most dogs and cats do well on a raw diet, but some prefer it slightly cooked and this can change with the season. Gipsy refuses to eat raw meat in the winter and likes me to add some grain, whereas in summer she likes her food raw and lean and will not eat grains at all. Raw food advocates claim that cooking destroys nutrients and this is true, but as a rule, our domestic animals are fed so well for such little effort, that a healthy animal gets more than enough. The loss of nutrients on lightly cooked meat is negligible and the digestibility and palatability of the food is increased, so cooking can be beneficial in some cases.

Of course, many animals seem to live perfectly well on commercially prepared food. However, an animal fed a natural diet has a much better balance in the stress account than one who is overburdened with toxins from a poor quality diet. Age, temperament, season, climate, health, all affect what a dog or cat chooses to eat and how he deals with the food he is given. People are amazed that even animals who wolf down anything will be discriminating once all their nutritional needs are met, and they are not faced with the same dish of kibble day in and day out.

Feeding choices for a cat or dog in order of preference:

- » Raw meat and bones
- » Home cooked food
- » Commercially prepared 'raw food diet'
- » Dried food that has meat as the main ingredient and contains no soy, wheat, chemical preservatives, flavouring/colourings.

Both cats and dogs, being hunters, digest their food better if a certain amount of effort has gone into obtaining it. So, the best time to feed a dog is when it returns from exercise, or play 'hide and seek' games with it before feeding. Cats who are housebound can have their food scattered for them so they have to spend some time tracking it down, or play hunting games with them before feeding times.

A final word on cats

By the time a cat is 12 weeks old she becomes highly suspicious of new food. She is unlikely to eat anything she hasn't tasted in this time or what her mother ate while nursing. It can be difficult to switch a cat who has always eaten dried food to a fresh diet, but with perseverance it is possible.

THE CHINESE PERSPECTIVE

When creating the correct diet for any individual, I also refer to Oriental principles of food as medicine. One of the building blocks of both Chinese and Ayurvedic medicine is diet. By adjusting an individual's diet, you assist the process of rebalancing the body and returning it to health.

The Rule of Fives

The Chinese view includes five temperatures, five climates, and five tastes. Each taste has an effect on the body, and you can balance the climates with the tastes. Individuals are constitutionally disposed towards one temperature or another, somewhere on the Hot (yang) or Cold (yin) scale.

If a constitutionally hot animal eats too much heating food, he will produce symptoms of heat, such as red inflamed skin, fever or excitability. To balance this, feed something cooling. The Chinese categorise food by taste and temperature, with each taste having a specific action on the body. A healthy diet will include all five tastes:

> » Sour (Wood) - stimulates the liver, controls diarrhoea and excessive perspiration
>
> » Bitter (Fire) – reduces fevers, stimulates digestion
>
> » Sweet (Earth) – aids digestion, neutralises toxins
>
> » Pungent (Metal) – improves circulation of Qi and Blood
>
> » Salty (Water) – softens hard nodules, including knotted muscles

Hot or Cold?

The temperature of foods can be categorised as either Yin (Cold) or Yang (Hot) but are further broken down into: Hot, Warm, Neutral, Cool, Cold.

The most important thing to consider from a Chinese perspective is the climate of the animal and his symptoms. The exterior climate is also a factor. On a very simplistic level, if you have a hot condition (redness of the skin, inflammation, excitability) avoid heating foods. If you have a cold condition (stiffness, arthritis, depression, soft nodules), feed foods that are heating and stimulant. Feed warming foods in winter, cooling foods in summer. Unless you are treating a specific problem, what you feed should add up to a neutral temperature, e.g. put a heating meat with a cooling grain.

FOUR KEY WORDS

Quality

The quality of a food is important, how it is produced from beginning to end affects it not only chemically, but energetically. Therefore, organic food raised lovingly and with respect for all, is ideal. But most importantly, food should be fresh.

Variety

Feeding a varied diet is also important. The body can become sensitised to anything if exposed to it too often, such as has happened with soy and wheat. Plus a varied diet is more likely to provide all the nutrients an animal needs.

Choice

As an extension to allowing animals to guide our use of essential oils, I always try to provide my animals with the choice to reject a foodstuff, or to eat something really strange, as long as I know it is not harmful. So, when feeding a dog I do not liquidise the vegetables, but grate or chunk, then lightly steam them, so he can pick around them if he chooses.

I do not mix additives into feed but allow my animals to pick and choose what they need. My animals, being used to having their nutritional needs fulfilled, will vary their diet from day to day, leaving behind perfectly good food if it does not suit them and only eating as much as they need.

Easy is right!

In an ideal world, everyone would feed their animal an unprocessed diet of organic origin, adjusted every day (or at least every week) to suit the changes in animal and weather conditions. In actuality, many people don't even cook for themselves. Why has pre-packaged food become so popular (apart from successful marketing)? Because it is convenient!

The diet must suit both animal and carer to be effective and often there will be some sort of compromise between the ideal and the practical. For instance, for reasons of practicality you may need to feed dried food as your dog's main diet, in which case, use a high quality food and add chicken wings, meaty bones, or raw liver a couple of times a week.

Stabled horses, fed on mass-produced hay and mixed cereals can be taken out in hand to graze the hedgerows or places where native plants are growing (this is also a great way to bond with your horse). If there is no access to herbage then feed dried herbs… A little creative thinking can go a long way.

The Climate of Food

Climate	Protein	Grains	Fruit and veg
Hot	Chicken fat, venison, lamb, smoked fish, trout.		Chilli pepper.
Warm	Salmon, tuna, chicken, turkey, beef, cheese, milk, egg yolk.	Oats.	Dates, ginger, cauliflower, green pepper, turnips.
Neutral	Egg whites, milk, pork, rabbit, chicken gizzard, sardines.	Brown rice, rye quinoa, corn.	Apricots, beetroot, broad beans, carrots, cauliflower, cabbage, peanuts, peas, plums, sweet potatoes, pears.
Cool	Duck.	Barley, wheat, millet.	Alfalfa, almonds, apples, broccoli, celery, spinach, salt, seaweed, turnip, watermelon.
Cold	Ice cream, mussels, tofu, yogurt.		Bean sprouts, cucumbers, lettuce, peppermint, tomato.

A word on vitamins, minerals and other food additives

Do you need to supplement a diet with vitamins and minerals? Some say you must, others say you shouldn't. It is true that heat destroys vitamins and minerals to a degree. Also, it is possible there are less vitamins and minerals in food because of poor agricultural practices. However, I believe a healthy animal will get enough of both if fed good fresh food.

Stressed animals absorb nutrients less efficiently, which can lead to an imbalance of minerals and subsequent problems. In which case I would consider using a supplement, as well as reducing stress. For instance, a lack of magnesium can contribute to nervous behaviour, supplementing with magnesium may then be appropriate in the short term until the body returns to balance.

I use supplements as a medicine and give them when they are needed. The other supplement I use regularly is oil, either herbal or vegetable, especially olive oil, coconut, flax or hemp seed.

Finally, the most common dietary problem – obesity

Overfeeding is one of the most common problems for domestic animals and is as much of an abuse as underfeeding. Over-eating leads to a wide range of diseases, especially heart problems and musculo-skeletal malfunction, but also bad temper. You must be especially careful with cats who can develop hepatic lipidosis, a potentially fatal disease, if they become ill or stop eating for any reason and lose weight rapidly. For the equine, the added stress of bearing excess weight as well as a rider often leads to lameness.

Barring any underlying illness, such as thyroid disease, the only reason an animal becomes fat is because there is more energy (food) going into the system than is being used. If you feed less and exercise more, the problem will dissolve (literally!). A healthy animal is lean, you should be able to feel his ribs under a light covering of flesh, if you cannot feel the ribs your animal is overweight.

In conclusion

By making simple changes to how we care for our animals, especially feeding them a species-specific diet, we reduce physiological stress and have healthier animals.

GLOSSARY OF TERMS

Amenorrhoea	Absence of menstruation
Anaemia	Deficiency in either quality or quantity of red blood corpuscles
Anaesthetic	Substance causing loss of feeling or sensation
Analgesic	Relieves pain without producing anaesthesia
Anaphrodisiac	Reduces sexual desire
Anodyne	Stills pain and quiets disturbed feelings
Antacid	Counteracts or neutralises acidity (usually in the stomach)
Anthelmintic	Destroys intestinal worms
Anti-allergenic	Relieves or controls allergic symptoms
Anti-anaemic	Prevents or cures anaemia
Anti-anxiety	Prevents or cures anxiety
Anti-arthritic	Prevents or cures arthritis
Antibacterial	Destroys bacteria or inhibits their growth
Anticatarrhal	Relieves inflammation of the mucous membranes in the head, and reduces the production of mucous.
Anticoagulant	Prevents or stops the blood clotting
Anticonvulsant	Stops, prevents or lessons convulsions/seizures
Antidepressant	Prevents or cures depression
Antiemetic	Reduces nausea/vomiting
Antifungal	Destroys or prevents the growth of fungi
Antihistamine	Used to treat allergies because it counteracts the effects of histamine such as inflammation, swelling, congestion, sneezing and itchy eyes.
Anti-inflammatory	Reduces inflammation
Anti-lactogenic	Reduces milk production
Anti-neuralgic	Relieves neuralgia (nerve pain), which is an acute, severe, intermittent pain that radiates along a nerve.
Antioxidant	Substance that prevents or slows oxidation. Research shows that some anti-oxidants can prevent cell damage.
Anti-parasitic	Kills or inactivates parasites
Antiphlogistic	Reduces inflammation
Antipruritic	Relieves itching
Antirheumatic	Relieves rheumatism
Antisclerotic	Prevents hardening of tissue

Anti-seborrhoea	Prevents the abnormal secretion and discharge of sebum, which gives the skin an oily appearance and forms greasy scales.
Antiseptic	Inhibits the growth and reproduction of microorganisms, when applied to the body it reduces the possibility of infection, sepsis or putrefaction.
Antispasmodic	Prevents/eases spasms or convulsions
Anti-sudorific	Prevents or inhibits sweating/perspiration
Antitoxic	Counteracts a toxin or poison
Anti-tussive	Inhibits the cough reflex helping to stop coughing
Antiviral	Inhibits growth of a virus
Aperient	Mildly laxative
Aphrodisiac	Increases sexual desire
Arthritis	Inflammation of joints
Astringent	Causes contraction of organic tissues, control of bleeding, styptic
Bactericidal	Kills bacteria
Calmative	Mildly sedative, relaxing
Cardio-tonic	Strengthens and invigorates the heart
Carminative	Reduces flatulence, settles digestive system
Cephalic	Referring to diseases affecting the head and upper part of the body. A remedy for disorders of the brain
Cholagogue	Stimulates secretion of flow of bile into duodenum
Choleretic	Stimulates the production of bile by the liver
Cicatrisant	Promotes formation of scar tissue and aids healing
Circulatory	Aids circulation of blood
Concrete	Waxy concentrated solid or semi-solid perfume material, prepared from previously live plant matter,
Damp	A Chinese bodily Climate that can lead to fungal infections, sluggishness, and fatty lumps.
Diaphoretic	Reduces fever by inducing sweating
Decongestant	Relieves congestion, usually by reducing the swelling of the mucous membranes in the nasal passages
Deficient	Lacking in energy, not functioning to optimal level of meridian systems
Deodorant	Masks or suppresses odours
Detoxicant	Removes toxins – substances which have a harmful chemical nature
Digestive stimulant	Stimulates digestion
Digestive tonic	Strengthens and invigorates digestion
Diuretic	Aids production of urine flow
Emmenagogue	Induces menstruation
Emollient	Softens, soothes and lubricates the skin
Energising	Invigorates and gives energy
Enuresis	Urinary incontinence
Euphoric	Exaggerated feeling of well being or elation
Excess	Too much energy causing an imbalance in a meridian system
Expectorant	Promotes clearing of chest/lungs
Febrifuge	Combats fever, antipyretic
Fortifying	Strengthening
Glandular tonic	Strengthens and invigorates the glands

Haemostatic	Stops bleeding
Heat	A Chinese bodily climate that can lead to inflammation, itching and excitability
Hepatic	Encourages healthy function of the liver,
Hormone-like	Acts like a hormone
Hydrosol/hydrolat	Also known as floral water, condensed water from distillation of aromatic plants
Hyperglycaemic	Having excessively high blood sugar
Hypoglycaemic	Having excessively low blood sugar
Hypertensive	Raises blood pressure
Hypo-uricemic	Breaks down uric acid
Hypotensive	Lowers blood pressure
Immune tonic	Strengthens and invigorates the immune system
Immunostimulant	Stimulates various functions or activities of the immune system
Infusion	Herbs steeped in liquid to extract soluble constituents
Insect repellent	Repels insects
Insecticide	Kills insects
Kidney tonic	Strengthens and invigorates the kidneys
Lactogenic	Enhances milk production
Laxative	Moves the bowels and aids digestion
Leukocyte-stimulant	Increases the production of leukocytes, which are white blood cells involved in fighting infections
Limbic system	A group of interconnected deep brain structures, common to all mammals, and involved in olfaction, emotion, motivation, behaviour and various autonomic functions.
Litholytic	An agent that dissolves urinary calculi (stones)
Meridian	The channels that distribute energy around the body according to Traditional Chinese Medicine
Meridian system	The organs, body parts, emotions and bodily functions that are connected to each meridian
Macerated oil	Infusion of herbs in vegetable oil
Mucolytic	Dissolves mucous
Nervine	Having a soothing effect on the nerves
Neurotonic	Strengthens and invigorates the nerves
Oestrogen-like	Has a similar effect on the body to that of oestrogen
Olfactory system	The parts of the body involved in sensing smell, including the nose and many parts of the brain
Pancreatic stimulant	Increases pancreatic activity
Parasiticide	Destroys parasites internally and externally
Pathogenic	Causing or producing disease
Pathological	Unnatural or destructive process on living tissue
Phlebotonic	Having a toning action on the veins
Purgative	Strongly laxative
Pyorrhoea	Bleeding or discharge of pus
Regenerative	Restores or revives tissue growth
Reproductive stimulant	Increases reproductive activity in the body
Restorative	Restores health or strength

Rubifacient	Causes redness of skin, possibly irritation
Sedative	Reduces excitability and calms the nerves
Sexual tonic	Strengthens and invigorates the sexual function
Smooth muscle relaxant	Relaxes the smooth muscles, which are muscles that contract without conscious control and are found in the walls of internal organs such as stomach, intestine and bladder
Soothing	Brings comfort or relief
Soporific	Sleep inducing
Stimulant	Increases physiological or nervous activity in the body; promotes activity, interest or enthusiasm
Stomachic	Promotes digestion or appetite
Styptic	Stops the flow of blood from wounds by contracting tissue or blood vessels
Sudorific	Produces sweat
Tincture	Alcoholic solution of some (usually vegetable) principle, used in medicine
Tonic	Strengthens and invigorates
Uterine tonic	Strengthens and invigorates the uterus
Vasodilator	Widens or dilates blood vessels
Vermifuge	Expels intestinal worms, anthelmintic
Vesicant	Causes blistering to skin, a counter-irritant by external application

RESOURCES AND REFERENCES

BIBLIOGRAPHY AND RECOMMENDED READING

Aromatics:

Aromatherapy for Healing the Spirit, Gabriel Mojay

Aromatherapy for Health professionals, Shirley Price and Len Price

Carrier Oils, Len Price, with Ian Smith and Shirley Price

Hydrosols, The Next Aromatherapy, Suzanne Catty

Medical Aromatherapy: Healing with Essential Oils, Kurt Schnaubelt

The Chemistry of Aromatherapeutic Oils, E.Joy Bowles

The Complete Guide to Aromatherapy, Salvatore Battaglia

The Encyclopedia of Essential Oils, Julia Lawless

Understanding Hydrolats: specific hydrosols for aromatherapy, Len & Shirley Price

The Clay Cure, Natural healing from the Earth, Ran Knishninsky

Animal care:

Down to Earth Natural Horse Care, Lisa Ross-Williams

Give Your Dog a Bone: The Practical Common Sense Way to Feed Dogs For a Long Healthy Life, Ian Billinghurst

Healthy Dogs, Your Loving Touch, Sherri Cappabianca

Natural Nutrition For Dogs & Cats: The Ultimate Diet, Kymythy Schultze

Wild Health, How animals keep themselves well and what we can learn from them, Cindy Engel

Chinese Medicine:

A Guide to Traditional Chinese Food Energetics, Daverick Leggett

Between Heaven and Earth, A guide to Chinese Medicine, Harriet Beinffield, L.Ac, Efrem Korngold, L.Ac., O.M.D.

Four Paws Five Directions, Cheryl Schwartz, DVM

The Web That Has No Weaver, Ted J. Kaptchuk O.M.D

Healing with Whole Foods, Paul Pitchford

ESSENTIAL OIL SUPPLIERS

USA

- » Ananda Aromatherapy, www.anandaapothecary.com
- » Aromatics International, www.aromaticsinternational.com
- » Eden Botanicals www.edenbotanicals.com
- » Floracopeia, www.floracopeia.com
- » Stillpoint Aromatics www.stillpointaromatics.com

Europe

- » Base Formula www.baseformula.com
- » Florihana, www.florihana.com
- » Kobashi, www.kobashi.com
- » Materia Aromatica, www.materia-aromatica.co.uk
- » Oshadhi www.oshadhi.com
- » Over the Edge Farm (Hydrosols) www.otefarm.eu
- » Norfolk Oils, www.neoils.com
- » The Wild Health Shop, www.thewildhealthshop.co.uk

ABOUT THE AUTHOR

Nayana Morag grew up in the UK in a large family of humans and animals, the perfect environment for learning about animal behaviour. By the age of 18 she had developed an interest in natural health and complementary medicines and started to travel widely, learning about everything from horse care to Hippocrates as she went.

In 1999 Nayana earned her *Certificate in Animal Aromatherapy and Touch for Health for Animals* and has been practising her art ever since. She also holds an *International Certificate in Aromatherapy*, through the *Pacific Institute of Aromatherapy*. She has a *Certificate in Systematic Kinesiology through T.A.S.K*, a *Post Graduate Certificate in Five Element Theory and Aromatic Energetics*, from *The Institute of Traditional Herbal Medicine and Aromatherapy*, and a *Master Herbalist Diploma* from *CoE*.

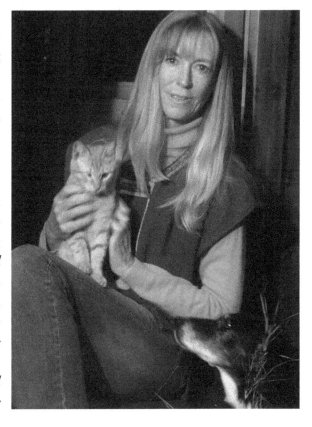

Over the years, Nayana has developed a system of animal wellness called *Animal PsychAromatica (APA)* that incorporates aromatics, *Traditional Chinese Medicine*, and reducing stress through management and diet. She offers online courses through the *Academy of Animal Wellness and Aromatics* at *www.essentialanimals.com*. Or you can learn from her in person at her home in Portugal, *www.otefarm.eu*.

CPSIA information can be obtained
at www.ICGtesting.com
Printed in the USA
BVHW060842071220
595088BV00001B/20